60-Second Secrets

www.60secondsecrets.com.au

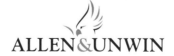

ALLEN&UNWIN

60-Second Secrets

to a **happy**, **healthy**, more **relaxed** you

Julie Maree Wood

ALLEN&UNWIN

First published in 2010

Allen & Unwin
83 Alexander Street
Crows Nest NSW 2065
Australia
Phone: (61 2) 8425 0100
Fax: (61 2) 9906 2218
Email: info@allenandunwin.com
Web: www.allenandunwin.com

Cataloguing-in-Publication details are available
from the National Library of Australia
www.librariesaustralia.nla.gov.au

ISBN 978 1 74237 209 9

Internal design and typesetting by Emily O'Neill
Printed in China at Everbest Printing Co. Ltd

10 9 8 7 6 5 4 3 2

Contents

Preface

In the time of our grandmothers, basic naturopathic practice and beliefs were part of the common lore. If you were ill, you took barley water, stayed in bed and nourished your body with easily digestible foods. If there was a cold wind, you kept your chest and throat protected and ventured out only if you had to. You took time to recover or convalesce from an illness. This commonsense approach to health was innate in our culture.

In these busy, frenetic times, we have lost much of this common lore and, as such, lost our connection to the healing power of foods and nature, of establishing balance in our everyday lives and becoming aware of what will truly bring us health and happiness.

A large part of practising naturopathy in these times is re-educating people about this lost knowledge or lore, of reconnecting them to the world around them, teaching them to listen to the natural rhythms of their bodies, and encouraging them to do small, simple things each day to keep them healthy and happy. I am a practising naturopath, yet still I sometimes get caught up in the whirlwind that is everyday life and forget my promise to myself to tend to my wellbeing a little each day. Some days I need to actually do, make or say something to keep this promise. On other days, I just need to think for a moment about how I am travelling, to check in with myself and my health.

It's easy to do but hard to remember.

I wrote this book to interrupt our everyday chaos and remind myself, and all of you, of what our grandmothers already knew—the secret to great health and happiness is to do one small thing each day to keep you feeling vital and alive.

Simple.

Introduction

Health is about more than just staying well. Being truly healthy is about being the most energetic, happy, positive, bright and balanced that you can be. It's about feeling great to be alive!

This book is a collection of simple secrets, big and small, that you can do, think about, make or practise throughout the year to bring you one step closer to becoming your best you. They are arranged according to the seasons and take only 60 seconds to read but the benefits can last a lifetime.

If the people I see in my clinic took a little secret time each day, they could feel fantastic and I would be out of business. Nagging symptoms such as exhaustion, poor skin, loss of vitality, fatigue, constipation, irritability and anxiety are common and can often be easily prevented or resolved if we just invested a moment or two every day.

Before you know it, your secret will be out and you'll be bouncing out of bed every morning!

In health and happiness,

Julie Maree Wood

Naturopath, nutritionist, mother of two

All of the entries contained within this book were written in good faith.

Before making any major changes to your diet or lifestyle please consider any allergies or health concerns you may have and consult a healthcare professional.

To my lovely husband Justin who reminds me of the secrets everyday and the three Lisas—Huck, Rischmiller and Reid—fantastic women, just like you, for whom I wrote this book.

A special thank you to Xavier, Charlie, Mum, Dad, Judy, Peter, the UK Woods, Franca Guarna, Jane Evans, Maggie Hamilton, Ann Lennox, Emma, Chris White and the great mums and teachers at St Joan of Arc.

The secrets

Spring

Summer

Autumn

Winter

Spring

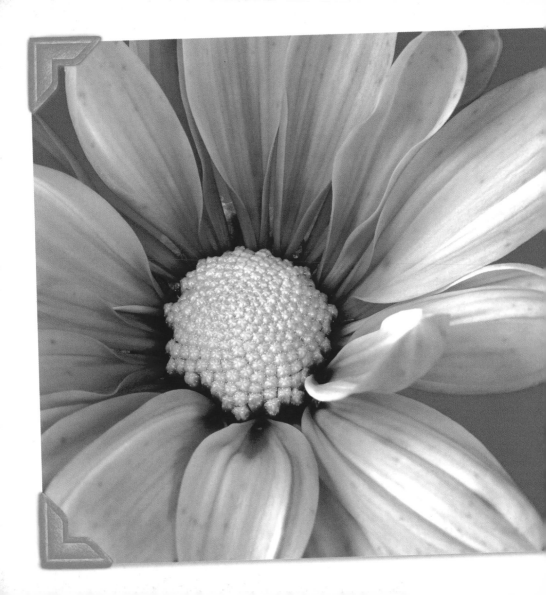

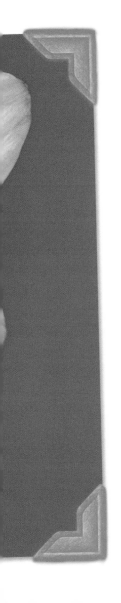

Spring, a busy season for nature. A time when the chill of winter fades and the warmth of summer begins to shine upon us.

The rain, heat, light and busy bees work together to give us the beautiful blooms and fruits of spring. The heady scent of jonquils and jasmine hang heavy on the breeze and the lilac jacarandas and vibrant cherry blossoms colour the landscape.

It's a time of new life and new beginnings, a time to feel invigorated and alive.

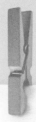

Spring diet

Spring is a beautiful time of year that is all about new life, renewed energy and re-energising ourselves after the winter chill. Time to change to the lighter diet of spring. Move slowly away from the heavy, well-cooked diet of winter and begin to eat warm salads and more fresh, uncooked foods as they come into season.
Focus on young plants, sprouts and fresh greens, all simply prepared.

Spring is the time to start to transition the body from the heaviness and hibernation of winter to the openness and light of the spring and summer months. Spring can be a blend of cool and hot days so mix warm vegetables and meats into your cold salads and eat stewed and raw fruits as you move into the more predictable warmer months.

Seasonal bikkies for smart cookies

Why not celebrate spring with some seasonal bikkies like these citrus drops?

Beat together 90 grams (3 ounces) of soft butter and ½ cup firmly packed brown sugar until pale. Add 1 lightly beaten egg and stir until combined. Add ¼ cup almond meal, ¼ cup wheatgerm, 1 tablespoon grated lemon rind, 1 tablespoon grated orange rind, 2 tablespoons LSA, ¾ cup wholemeal plain flour and ½ cup wholemeal self-raising flour. Stir to combine, adding a drop of water if required. Roll teaspoonfuls into balls, place on a lined baking tray and flatten with a fork. Bake in a moderate oven for 12–15 minutes.

Everybody loves a good bikkie. Life is not about denying ourselves the pleasures it offers, it's about enjoying them in moderation. These citrus drops are only bite size and are loaded with lots of nutritional goodies, so if you're going to have a biscuit treat, they are a good choice! LSA is a mixture of ground linseeds, sunflower seeds and almonds, available from any health food shop.

Smells of spring

Bring some spring into your home today. Buy or make a spring blend with essential oils. Blend 3 drops each of bergamot, petitgrain and tangerine essential oils and burn in your oil burner to fill your home with the fresh scent of spring.

Smell is a lovely sense to stimulate at the beginning of this beautiful season. Blend as you go or make a small bottle of the blend to use throughout the spring. If you have only one or two of the oils, it will work just as well.

Springtime punch

Spring is here but still some of the bugs of winter are lingering. Have a dose of this springtime punch today to keep on top of them.

Juice 1 red, seeded capsicum and 1 tomato. Stir in half a finely sliced, small red deseeded chilli.

Add a squeeze of lemon juice, then strain.

Have a sip to check the heat and then drink it down.

Capsicums and chillies have three times as much vitamin C as oranges, so this juice is like a vitamin C blast.

Home spa

Your body has been hiding under all of those jumpers through winter, so let's get it ready for your skimpy summer wardrobe. This is a five-minute home spa treatment to do in your own bathroom today.

Mix together 5 dessertspoons quick oats, 2 teaspoons salt, 1½ teaspoons ground rice, 2 dessertspoons vegetable or almond oil and 4 drops lavender essential oil. Press it down in a glass jar. Using a small amount at a time, rub it over the entire body. Rinse off and repeat each week so you'll be smooth and silky for summer.

The grittiness of the oats, rice and salt work to slough off dead skin cells and feed our new summer skin.

Nose breathing

Do some pranayama breathing today. Sit comfortably on a chair. Close your eyes. Still your mind. Place a thumb over one nostril and breathe in through the other. Move your thumb to the other nostril and breathe out. Breathe in and out, alternating nostrils, for about five minutes. If you feel short of breath, breathe through your mouth until you are relaxed again and then resume the nose breathing.

Breathing delivers oxygen to all of our organs. Breathing exercises, or pranayama, are one of the five principles of yoga. Learning to control our breathing works on both our mind and body. It can help us to relax, recentre and give our organs the vital oxygen they need. It is a wonderful health tool.

Smudge stick for spring

Freshen the air, warm the atmosphere and clear unpleasant smells and energies from your home with a spring smudge stick (you will repeat this in the autumn).

Traditionally, sage and sweetgrass are used but a bunch of mixed fresh woody herbs such as thyme, lavender or rosemary will work just as well. Tie the bunch together with some pure cotton string and leave to dry out for a few weeks. When the bunch is dry, carefully light it. The herbs will slowly begin to smoulder and smoke. Gently wave the smudge stick around the room. Allow the smoke to transform the air. Once the smell of the herbs has filled the room, extinguish the smudge stick.

Smudging is a powerful cleansing technique from the Native North American tradition. Always keep a close eye on your smudge stick to ensure that the herbs only smoulder with no flame. To extinguish the smudge stick, dip it into sand and then trim the burnt ends.

Rub the stress away

The working day has finished and you finally get to sit down and relax. Keep a small bottle of scented massage oil next to your chair, for a five-minute evening hand massage. Sandalwood, rose, lavender, patchouli and German chamomile essential oils are all wonderful for soothing a stressed mind and body.

Blend them with a good quality base oil such as jojoba. Massage the entire hand, focusing on the fleshy joint area between the thumb and index finger.

The area between the thumb and index finger is a stress harbour for many people. Gently massaging the area can help to relax the body and mind and ease headaches and tension. Don't use too much pressure—just a firm but gentle massage will do the trick.

Holiday plans

Start to plan a holiday today.
It doesn't have to be a five-star
extravaganza, just something that suits
your budget.
Set the date so you can look forward to it.

Remember when you were a child and you always had
something to look forward to. We seem to lose this
somewhere along the way and when we become adults,
life can become a grind. Setting dates and things to
look forward to can give us a sense of time, purpose
and satisfaction.

The ace of hearts

Love your heart today.
Feed it with foods rich in potassium, calcium and essential fatty acids. This means salmon, sardines, butternut, seaweed, sunflower oil, tofu, linseed oil, almonds, broccoli, green leafy vegetables, avocado, banana, pecans and cashews.
Eat foods containing good fats such as avocado, nuts, good quality oils and deep-sea fish.
Take a short walk at lunchtime to get your blood moving, your heart pumping and your muscles working.

The cornerstones of good heart health are eating foods rich in the heart's vital nutrients, drinking lots of water, choosing good fats not bad, exercising and maintaining a healthy weight.

Be free

Play your favourite song.
Dance like nobody is watching.

Remember that wonderful carefree feeling you had as a child? You were in the moment, enjoying yourself and dreaming your dreams. Music is a great way to reconnect and bring yourself into the moment, to regain that carefree abandon, banish the stresses of the day and free your spirit.

Beans means health

Your superfood for today is beans.
This means broad beans, French beans, stringless beans, soy beans, black beans, any beans.
Eat at least two serves today.
Be daring and try a variety you haven't tried before.
Have them in a soup, a stew, a curry, on their own, or just drain a can of them and toss them through your salad.

Beans are high in folate, potassium, magnesium, B vitamins, protein and fibre, making them good for the heart, the digestive system and for boosting energy.

Eye lift

Check your eyes today. Are they sore and puffy? Any dark circles underneath? How about an easy ten-minute eye lift?

Choose one of these:
- Cut two slices of raw potato. Place one on each eye and lie down for ten minutes.
- Grate some cucumber and some potato. Soak two cottonwool pads in the mixture and refrigerate until cold. Place one pad on each eye and lie down for ten minutes.
- Mix together 1 teaspoon natural yoghurt and 1 teaspoon honey. Carefully apply to the skin around the eyes and leave on for ten minutes. Rinse off.

Dark circles under the eyes can be hereditary, due to lack of sleep, stress of the eye muscles from burning the midnight candle, kidney issues or a sign of allergies. The circles are made worse by smoking, poor diet and too many stimulants such as coffee.

Ver equinox

Look up on the internet the date of this year's Ver
(from the Latin *ver* meaning spring) equinox.
Mark it in your diary.
Plan a small ceremony to welcome the equinox as it is
the first true day of spring.

For thousands of years humans have followed the movements of the
planets and the ebb and flow of the seasons, the rhythms of the Earth.
Reconnecting to these rhythms connects us to our spirit and our higher
sense of being. The seasons change according to the movement of the
Earth and sun, not the calendar. For this reason, celebrate the equinox
and welcome spring for another year.

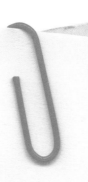

Turn off autopilot

Be mindful today.
What does the water in the shower really feel like on your skin? How does that strawberry taste? What does it feel like when your child is giving you a hug?

Making yourself connect with the present and being mindful of its details can uncover the beauty that can be found in everyday life. If you have trouble connecting with the present, watch a young child. This is their natural state, which is why they have such a wonderful love of life.

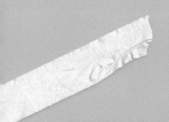

Natural first aid

Add one more cheap, effective remedy to your natural first aid kit today: the tissue salt Ferr Phos. It's just the thing if you have any inflammation, redness or throbbing, or at the first sign of a cough or respiratory infection.
Start dosing, as per the instructions on the label, at the first sign of symptoms.

Tissue salts are simple homeopathic preparations that are safe for all the family to use. They help the body to restore its natural balance and are an excellent tool to use before reaching for the stronger medicines. Always consult your healthcare professional if symptoms persist.

Essential kitchen garden

Spring brings with it the wonderful opportunity to breathe life back into your kitchen herb garden. For a basic herb garden, plant some parsley, dill and mint.
If you like to cook Indian food, put in some curry and chillies.
For Italian food fans, plant some oregano, basil and thyme and for those who like Thai some Vietnamese mint and Thai basil will do the trick.

Herbs are easy to grow—even for those without a green thumb—and bring dishes alive when they are used straight from the garden. Ensure they get lots of sun, water and a little love and they will give you wonderful meals through the warmer months.

Brain surge

Let's banish that 3 p.m. afternoon slump today.
Don't reach for a coffee.
Pick some rosemary from your garden or buy a bottle
of rosemary essential oil and keep it on your desk.
When you feel the slump on its way, take a few
deep breaths of the rosemary and have a
large glass of water.
You will feel it clear your head as you become more
focused and aware, ready to face the afternoon.

Rosemary has a wonderful stimulating effect on the nervous system.
It helps to stimulate sensory perception and memory and can also help
to alleviate tension and headache.

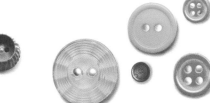

Memory music

Choose a song that was once one of your favourites.
Sit for five minutes and listen to the track.
Allow it to take you back to a wonderful memory.
Remember how you felt.
Hold on to this feeling after the song finishes.
Keep it with you for the day.

Music can help us reclaim memories, change our perspective, or lift our mood and being away from the everyday. It is a powerful tool that can be used any time to meet our physical, psychological, emotional, cognitive or social needs.

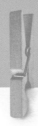

Feel loved

Sit and breathe for a few minutes and allow a sense of peace and self-acceptance to fill your heart.
If it leaves, invite it back and stay with the feeling.
Imagine you are in the arms of someone who truly loves you.
Keep this feeling with you for today.

Focused breathing has been used in the relaxation and healing arts for thousands of years. It can reduce heart rate, oxygen consumption and blood pressure, and so relax and rebalance the body, mind and spirit.

One-pot wonder

Make an addition to your first aid kit today.
Add a pot or tube of calendula cream.
It is a natural wonder.
You can use it on burns, dry skin, itchy areas, abrasions, small cuts, athlete's foot, anything that needs to be soothed and healed.
It will become your first aid one-pot wonder.

Calendula officinalis is the botanical name for those lovely bright orange flowers, sometimes called marigolds. It has wonderful healing properties, being anti-inflammatory, antiviral and wound healing. (Make sure you're using Calendula, not any other type of marigold.)

Dairy-free day

Make today a dairy-free day.
Replace your latte with a soy latte, use juice on
your cereal and have some fresh fruit or nuts
instead of yoghurt.

Dairy is a staple in the Western diet. Cutting a regular food such as dairy
from your diet for a time can move you out of your comfort zone and
inspire you to try new foods, thereby broadening your diet. It is a great
way to take off your blinkers and give you a fresh look at foods you may
never have considered.

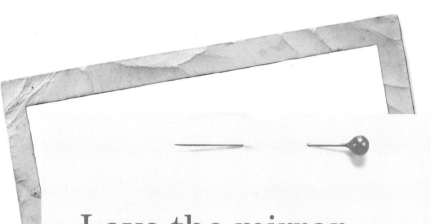

Love the mirror

Each time you wash your hands today, look up into the mirror, smile and tell yourself, 'I'm gorgeous'.

So often we are unnecessarily hard on ourselves.
Use this day to remind yourself that you are a unique, gorgeous person. There are many people in your life who see it every day. Today is your day to see it.

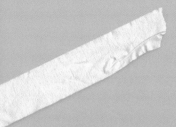

Tummy tuck

'Strong stomach, strong back.'
Whenever you see the colour red today,
pull in your abdominal muscles and hold them tight
for a count of ten.
Repeat the movement three times each time.

The abdominal muscles are the only front muscles supporting the back.
When they are weak we can suffer from, or exacerbate, back problems.
You don't need to go to the gym to have a trim tummy. Just exercise
them throughout the day when you are sitting, standing or walking.
Using a colour to trigger the exercise is a great way to remind you
to do it.

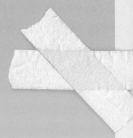

Fresh is best

Spring is the time to plant your herb garden in time for summer.
Start to plan it today.
Basil, thyme, oregano, parsley, mint, coriander, dill and chervil are all easy to grow. Just plant them in a place with lots of sunshine and water regularly.

Fresh herbs have myriad medicinal and nutritional properties. Having them fresh in your garden ensures that they are packed with nutrients and other goodies when you use them. The smell, touch and taste of the fresh herbs also inspire your appetite and desire for good, fresh, healthy food.

Resolve an issue

Choose an issue.
Begin with a small one.
Work out three things you could do today
to resolve the issue.

Unresolved issues can sit within us and wreak havoc with our health
and wellbeing. Sometimes we just need to take the bull by the
horns and resolve them one by one. Begin with small ones and
work up to the larger issues. For the larger ones, we may need to
speak to a professional to get some help in moving forward and
that's OK. Go online to find a reputable counsellor. Each state has
a counsellor's association with a site listing registered counsellors.
Our emotional health is intrinsically linked to our physical health,
so resolving emotional issues is pivotal to good health.

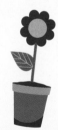

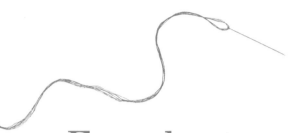

Free de-stress

We don't always have time to sit, clear our minds and relax, so, if you have a busy day ahead, try some soothing background music to de-stress you.
The internet is loaded with sites that offer free meditation and relaxation music.
Have a trawl around, find what you like and download it. Play it throughout the day to maintain a calm, relaxing energy in your home, car or workspace.

The internet is filled with gems. Type 'free meditation music' into Google, or your preferred search engine, and numerous sites will come up. Choose a reputable one such as The Meditation Society of Australia, where you know the music is legally on the net and the artists have agreed to its free download.

Spring clean your passages

The spring sun is shining, the birds are singing and the flowers are blooming. If you are a hayfever sufferer, this means the pollens and grasses are killing your nose! Before you pop a pill today, try clearing your passages naturally with some salted water.

You can use a traditional netti pot or a commercial product such as Fess.

Either way, the saline solution will get up your nose and clear your passages and sinuses without the need for drugs, removing the pollens and other irritants that are driving you crazy.

Nasal irrigation has been used by ayurvedic and yoga practitioners in India for hundreds of years. It clears the sinuses, makes breathing easier, can help to reduce the chances of any infection spreading, is cheap, easy and has no nasty side-effects.

Write it off

Put a small notepad and pen next to your bed today for those times when nagging thoughts and 'to do' lists keep going through your mind as you try to fall asleep. Write down everything so you clear your mind and drift off to sleep.

Good, sound sleep is vital to our health and wellbeing. An overactive mind at bedtime is a key factor in insomnia. Writing down nagging thoughts will take the burden from your mind and leave you in a state of calm, which is conducive to restful sleep.

Movie star hair and nails

Give your hair and nails a Hollywood makeover today.
Start with the inside by feeding them with foods rich in silica,
such as barley, oats, root vegetables and wholegrain cereals.
To naturally highlight dark hair, shampoo it, then rinse with
diluted lemon juice. To give it a shine, rinse with tea of
parsley, sage or rosemary. To naturally highlight fair hair,
shampoo it, then rinse with a strong tea of chamomile.
To give it a shine, rinse with a yarrow or calendula tea.

Silica is fundamental in the building and linking of collagen and other
connective tissue and so is vital for healthy hair and nails. Many of the more
expensive shampoos and conditioners contain it to give your hair an instant
boost. Increasing it in your diet will give you a much more lasting result.

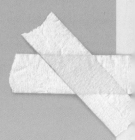

Liver lover

Spring is the time to attend to your liver.
When the liver is working efficiently, you will find yourself calm, decisive and able to cope with the stresses of life. Overindulgence in food and drink can lead to a sluggishness of the liver and a blockage of chi (life energy) and imbalance. To gently cleanse and support the liver, have the juice of half a lemon in some warm water in the morning. Use a straw to drink it to protect your teeth from the lemon's acid. Peppermint tea, cabbage, watercress, beetroot, carrot, kale, endive, rocket, radish and grapefruit are all great foods to support and nurture the liver.

The liver really is an extraordinary organ and one that needs a little periodic TLC. Cutting down on alcohol, eating liver friendly foods, and reducing artificial and processed foods will give your liver well-deserved R&R.

Drink smart

If you are looking to lose some weight, think about how much alcohol you drink today.
There are some simple ways to cut down the calories while still enjoying a tipple.
Have a white wine spritzer instead of a full glass of wine, or a light beer or a shandy instead of a full-strength beer.
Have a glass of mineral water between each drink.

Alcohol is riddled with calories and undoes the good work of many ardent dieters. Think of a glass of wine or beer as a piece of apple pie with cream. It may be just the motivation you need to stick to your weight-loss plan.

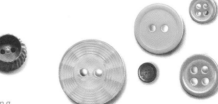

Complement your compliments

Take a little extra time to get ready today.
Make sure you look a bit special.
You are sure to receive some compliments.
Your task today is to practise receiving them graciously
and believe them.
If you hear a 'You look great today', how about replying with
a 'Well thank you very much', 'Thanks, I feel really good today'
or you could really go to town with a 'Yeah, I'm a fox!'.

Why do we find it so hard to take and believe a compliment? Too often we dismiss them with an off-hand remark. When people take the time to give you a compliment, they mean it. Take it on board, and the next time you look in the mirror, repeat the compliment to yourself. It is a great way to boost your self-esteem.

Natural mood lifter

We all have days when we are on edge, irritable and stressed. It may result in a headache, tight shoulders or just a very cranky you. Get some of the tissue salt Kali Phos, the Nerve Nutrient, today and take it next time one of those cranky days comes along. It is great for helping to ease nervous tension, irritability, low mood and tension-related headaches.

Start dosing, as per the instructions on the label, at the first sign of symptoms.

In the early nineteenth century, Doctor W.H. Schuessler, a German chemist and physicist, discovered tissue salts or minerals and found that an imbalance in any of these minerals could lead to illness or disease. As a result, he developed homeopathic tissue salts that could be used for common ailments and symptoms.

Gaze into your eyes

Have a good look into your eyes today.
Focus on the iris, the coloured part of your eye.
Is the outer rim of the iris nice and sharp or does it have a dark smudged line around it?
If there is a dark line around it, start daily dry skin brushing, get regular fresh air and gentle sunshine, and drink lots of water to help flush out your system.

Many naturopaths use iridology, a study of the iris, to get a snapshot of a person's state of health. Each part of the iris corresponds to an area of the body. The outer rim of the iris, where the iris colour joins the sclera, or white of the eyeball, corresponds to the skin. A dark smudged line around the edge of the iris is called a scurf rim and indicates that the skin is not clearing itself well and needs some attention.

Flower power

Buy or pick some fresh flowers today.
Put them in a vase in a spot you walk past regularly.

Fresh flowers bring a beautiful energy to a space. They are especially uplifting to a home if you live alone. It doesn't have to be a dozen red roses, just an inexpensive bunch from the supermarket or a few daisies from the garden will do the trick and keep your budget intact.

TLC for TMJ

The TMJ, or tempero mandibular joint, is the joint at
either end of your jaw, just in front of your ears.
Give it a stretch today with some simple exercises.
Put your tongue on the roof of your mouth and open
your mouth wide. Breathe in and count to five, then
breathe out and count to five.
Release and repeat five times.
Now make a fist and place it under your chin. Use
your fist to gently press your jaw closed and, at the
same time, use your jaw muscles to try to open your
mouth. Hold this and count to five. Repeat five times.
Finally, place a finger on each TMJ and gently rotate
it to massage and relax the area.

The TMJ is a common place for us to store stress and tension, making
the area feel tight and sore. Stretching and exercising will help to
loosen it and keep it relaxed.

Community chest

Make some community connections today.
When you pick up some milk at the shops, ask
the shopkeeper's name and have a quick chat.
Keep your head up when you walk home
from buying the paper and say 'Hi' to the
neighbours.
Give people a nod and hello on the stairs or
in the lift.
It will brighten their day and lift your spirits.

As humans, we are pack animals and have a great desire to
be connected to others. We have family and friends but we
can also be connected to the community. Knowing your local
shopkeepers and neighbours is a great way to broaden your
connections to the larger world beyond your front door.

Taking the sting from the bee

Bees love spring. It is their busiest time of year. Buy some homeopathic Apis from your health food shop before tiptoeing through the tulips this spring. Keep it handy and take a dose immediately if you get stung.

Apis mellifica is a homeopathic remedy used for bites and stings. It quickly settles the sharp pain of a bee sting. You will see the red line of the sting stop in its tracks if you take it immediately. Dose regularly as per the instructions on the pack. Apis is not a substitute cure for people with bee sting allergies. If you have an allergy to bee stings, follow your usual procedure.

Berry healthy

The superfood for today is blueberries. Buy some fresh or frozen today and use them in a milkshake, smoothie, dessert, fruit salad or on their own.

Blueberries are rich in many vitamins and minerals, including vitamins C and K, and manganese. The antioxidants in blueberries protect our cells from damage and can help to keep us happy and well.

Head traffic jam

It may be the pollens, it may just be a very long 'to do' list, but if you are feeling like there is a traffic jam in your head today, take five minutes and give yourself a steam inhalation. It will make the rest of your day much for enjoyable and productive.

Use two drops of one of these essential oils:

- Rosemary—to clear the mind and help you concentrate.
- Peppermint—to uplift, refresh and clear the mind.
- Lavender—to calm and balance a worried mind.

For a steam inhalation, tie your hair back and wash your face. Carefully pour 1 litre (1¾ pints) of boiling water into a bowl or saucepan on a heatproof non-slip mat on a table. Add your essential oil blend, put your face 20–30 centimetres (8–8½ inches) away from the water, cover your head with a towel or large cloth and breathe deeply and relax. Stay there for about ten minutes. Then wash your face clean with tepid water.

Volunteer your time

If you have some spare time or are looking for more structure and connection in your life, do some research on volunteering today.
There are many local charities and not-for-profit organisations in your area that would greatly value your contribution and compassion.

Volunteering is a wonderful way to bring a greater meaning to our lives. It brings with it a sense of connection and being needed, and opens up a new circle of friends.
It also gives us a new perspective on our being when we see others in need.

Boost your vital energy

Yellow is the colour to boost vital energy.
Bring some into your life today.
It may be something you wear, a flower you pick, a cup
you drink from or, if you are feeling really adventurous, a
wall you paint!
Bring out the yellow and feel your vital energy respond
and your creativity blossom.

In colour therapy, yellow energises the muscles.
It works with our mental capacity and can help with the creation of thoughts.
Being connected with the third chakra, near our solar plexus, yellow can raise
our vital energy making us feel more connected and alive.

Clean and clear

It is spring and there is no better time to clear out old clutter.
Clear out a cupboard a week, giving all that you no longer use to charity.

Detoxing has become a fashionable term. It is actually a very old naturopathic tradition. These days, detox focuses on the body alone and yet, for it to be truly effective, we need to give everything a regular clear out. Body, mind and spirit all benefit. Clearing out the clutter and rubbish in your environment is a great way to detox your space and allow you to move forward with a clear, calm and centred mind and being. What is your trash may well be someone else's treasure.

Reconnecting

Have a think about this today.
What is your place of spiritual connection?
Is it a traditional church building with a minister?
Is it sitting quietly in your favourite chair for five minutes?
Is it spending time with your roses in the garden?
What gives you a feeling of peace and happiness?
Whatever it is, think about how much time you spend there.
Could you find some time to spend there today?

We are all so busy, but it is often the simplest of things that can make us feel
happy and help to slow our life down. When we recognise what it is that makes
us feel happiest and most satisfied, it is amazing how we can find the time to
spend in that place. It need only be five minutes a day, but it will make a
world of difference.

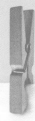

Buzz off naturally

Mosquitoes love the warmer months.
Before you reach for the chemical repellents, take some time today to mozzie-proof your house.
Check that there is no stagnant water in the gutters, ponds or pet bowls. Make sure your fly screens are intact and patch any holes. Rig up mosquito nets over the beds, especially the beds of those who the mozzies particularly love (there's often one person they love to bite). Buy a cheap fly swat to knock them down if they do get into the house.
Lavender, eucalyptus, tea tree and citronella essential oils are all fantastic natural repellents. Combine them in a clean spray bottle to mist the house or spray over yourself.

There are simple, natural things you can do to protect yourself and your family from mozzies. It is important to do as mosquitoes are carrying more and more nasty diseases.

Salty massage

Run a warm bath.
Sit on the edge and mix together a handful of sea salt and
enough bath water to make a paste.
Massage the paste all over your body, from your neck down to
the soles of your feet, using small circular movements.
Then soak in the bath for fifteen minutes.

Used externally, salt increases circulation, exfoliates the skin and is
stimulating to the body. It is a fantastic detoxifier and can be a great way to
stop an oncoming cold or flu in its tracks. If you suffer from haemorrhoids
or varicose veins, add another cup of salt to the bath water before you
soak as it will help to contract the veins. If you suffer from high or low
blood pressure, any heart conditions or have any broken skin, don't use this
bathing technique.

Spot checks

Do regular spot checks on your tension hot spots today.
Do you clench your jaw, grind your teeth, tighten your
shoulders, get a knot in your stomach?
Find the hot spot, relax it and breathe deeply, allowing
the tension to dissolve.

We get into habits of carrying tension and
stress in particular areas of our bodies.
Over time, these can cause stiffening and
problems in that area.

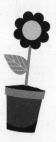

Emotional health check

Look at the list of Bach flowers below and see which apply to how you are feeling.
Buy the remedy that best suits you and begin to use it today; 4 drops, four times a day until finished.

- Cherry plum for irrational fear and thoughts
- Red chestnut for anxiety and feeling fear for others
- White chestnut for persistent worries, internal arguments and chatter
- Olive for burnout or exhaustion
- Mustard for depression, gloom or melancholy
- Gorse for hopelessness, chronic depression or pessimism
- Holly for envy, jealousy, anger, bitterness or hatred
- Crab apple for self-disgust or self-loathing
- Larch for a lack of self-confidence
- Mimulus for fear of known things
- Aspen for general fear

Bach flower remedies are made from the essence of flowers. They are similar to homeopathic medicines and work to gently promote healing in the body.

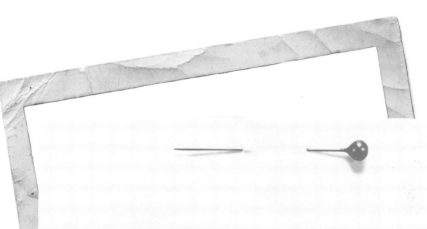

Quality time

Organise yourself, your children, nieces, nephews or grandchildren and a pile of books on your bed and read with them for an hour.

Children have a beautiful, pure energy. They are wonderful to spend time with and they love our time more than anything else. An hour reading will slow the frantic pace of your lives and connect you all.

Walk the walk

Today is an all-walking day.
You may have to drive the car to work and home, but park it there and walk for the rest of the day.
Walk up the stairs, walk to school, walk to sport, walk to coffee, walk to the shops and go for a big walk at lunchtime.

It's spring, so get outside and get some of that beautiful spring energy into you. Walking is a great way to do it. It will lift your energy and motivation, clear your mind and burn off a few of those extra winter calories you may have collected.

Back yourself

Think about your back today.
When you are carrying groceries, picking up children or working at the computer, how are you holding your back? Is it straight and strong?
Do you give it a rest at regular intervals?
What can you do to reduce the stress you put on it?
Not carrying too many heavy things at once, lifting correctly, adjusting the computer screen—all of these things can help avoid a sore, tired back.

Back pain can creep up on us and be debilitating. Just being aware of how we use our back and sometimes making small adjustments to the way we do things can make a huge difference in the long term.

Gossip no more

Make a pact with yourself not to gossip today.
Don't participate in it or listen to it.
You'll feel better about yourself and your energy will be more positive and balanced.

We all know that feeling we get when we know someone is gossiping about us. It is a terrible knot we get in our stomach and a burning feeling in our face. Even the most annoying people are hurt by gossip. Rather than wasting your energy on meaningless gossip, use your energy to improve your own life or help others who may need your assistance and don't need people gossiping about them.

Cheesy feet

If someone in your home has stinky feet,
today is the day to deal with them.
It's easy.
Get out your Epsom salts.
Pour half a cup of them into a footbath
and add some warm water.
Cheesy feet need to soak in the water
for fifteen minutes.
Problem solved.

The Epsom salts will deodorise the feet, with the pleasant
side-effect of relaxing the person soaking them. Perfect.

Building your creative energy

Your creative energy drives your willpower, your power of thought, gives you a presence, nourishes your being and is a vital part of conception.
It is strengthened by any form of stillness and by connecting with your higher, more spiritual self.
The best way to top it up is sound, uninterrupted sleep and meditation or any form of stillness.

Think of a pregnant woman or new mother. Many complain of 'baby brain'. They get muddled, confused and forgetful. This is due to a natural depletion in their creative energy as conceiving and birthing use a very concentrated form of this type of energy.

Tea plus one

For every cup of tea you have today, have an extra glass of water.

The caffeine in tea dehydrates the body and increases the need for water. Using your tea as a reminder to have a glass of water can be a great way to ensure you drink enough to stay hydrated and fresh.

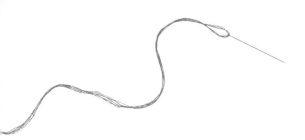

Just be silly

Remember when you were a child and you laughed so hard, you forgot what you were laughing about?
Afterwards you felt great.
There is something fantastic to learn there.
Do something silly today.
Don't leave the front door wide open or lock the keys in the car, do something frivolous and silly, like you would have done every day when you were a child.
Walk in the rain, jump in a puddle, race your partner to the front gate, jump on the bed, go on.

Kick the serious habit and just be silly. It feels great and lightens the load.

Ditch the itch

Is someone in your house itchy?
When all the spring grasses and pollens abound,
itchy skin often results.
Pop some urtica cream into your first aid kit today,
ready for the spring itch.
It can also be rubbed into the skin to help ease the
aches and pains of arthritis.

Urtica dioca, or stinging nettle, has long been used to treat itching,
pain and many other ailments. It was one of the nine plants in the pagan
Anglo-Saxon 'Nine Herbs Charm' recorded in the tenth century.
It will become an inexpensive, invaluable component of your natural
first aid kit.

Ponder this

Test run a new way of thinking today.
Instead of thinking about your body in terms of performance,
think about it in terms of how it feels.
How do you feel at your core?
Does your energy feel blocked anywhere?
Place your hands on where you feel blocked, sad or
unbalanced.
Close your eyes.
Breathe in and out.
Visualise the energy moving freely again.

Often, recognising a block in our energy and releasing it can be enough to
keep it moving freely. This is energetic self-healing. Energetic healers, such as
reiki, kinesiology, crystal therapy and acupuncture practitioners, work to clear
our energetic fields and keep things moving. They believe that when there is
stagnation in the movement of energy around the body, disease and illness
can develop.

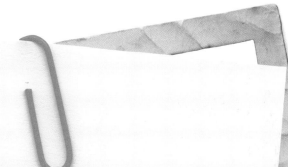

Natural food

The growing season is here.
Plant a little salad garden today.
You can use a mixture of lettuces—rocket, radicchio, mizuna, cos—and some salad herbs like dill, oregano, chives and basil.
Before you know it, you will have fresh, organic salads on your doorstep to last you through the warmer months.

Organic fresh food can be expensive and difficult to find. A small salad pot or garden is easy to grow and maintain, and will save you time and money. With an abundance of them, you will eat loads of nutritious salads throughout the spring and summer.

A medicinal spring clean

Take out your medicines and supplements today.
Now take five minutes to do some research on them and
check their use-by dates.
When was the last time you had them reviewed by your
doctor or healthcare professional?
Get on the net and look up the side-effects for each of
your medicines.
If you have any of the side-effects, note them in your diary
and have a chat to your doctor or healthcare professional
next time you visit them.

Over time, we can build up quite a collection of medicines and supplements
and forget to look at them and assess them as a whole. It is good practice to
have them regularly reviewed by a professional and to know the potential
side-effects and other problems they can cause.

New food phobic?

Be courageous today and try a food you have never tried before.
It may be a wedge of tofu, some legumes, a slice of wholegrain bread, anything new that is healthy and whole.

Get out of a food rut by opening yourself up to trying new foods. Variety is the simple key to good nutrition as different foods have different nutritional strengths and weaknesses.

Slow down life

Are you always rushing, with a million things running through your mind, constantly worrying, have no patience and just cannot find time for yourself?
That describes many of us.
It's so hard to slow life down and find a little time for ourselves.
Next time you are at the health food shop or chemist, pick up the Australian Bush Flower Essence Calm and Clear and keep it in your handbag.

Flower essences are a part of vibrational medicine and have been used in ancient Egypt, as well as India, Asia, Europe and South America, for thousands of years. You may already know the English Bach flower essences such as Rescue Remedy. Calm and Clear is also a flower essence preparation but it is made from only native Australian flowers and is part of the Australian Bush Flower Essences range.

Juice it

Buy or make vegetable juice today.
Be adventurous. Try something new.
Carrot is great for the eyes and liver.
Celery is good for the kidneys.
Ginger helps to break down mucus.
Parsley gives you a great iron boost.
Beetroot loves the liver.

Vegetable juices are an excellent way to boost your diet, giving you a burst of vitamins, minerals and phytonutrients. The phytonutrients in these fabulous juices help you to fight allergies, inflammation and free radicals, and boost the immune system. They are vital for good health.

Play up

Play hide and seek with your children, grandchildren, or nephews or nieces.

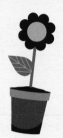

Playing with children connects us with a wonderful part of ourselves. It can make us feel free and forget our adult worries and problems. Children love the care and attention of adults, particularly those that are most important to them. A game of hide and seek is a win-win situation, no matter who wins the game.

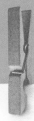

Chemical assault

Take a step in reducing the number of chemicals in your home today.
Get rid of your synthetic room sprays and deodorisers and buy all-natural alternatives or make your own.
Buy a spritzer bottle from the supermarket and three-quarters fill it with filtered water.
Add 5 drops each of lavender and lemon essential oils. Each time you use it, shake it first and then spray it liberally around the house to keep it feeling and smelling fresh and alive.

We are exposed to thousands of synthetic chemicals each day in the modern world. The more chemicals we can reduce in our home environment, the better.

Yoga time

How about combining your relaxation time
and your exercise time?
Use the internet to do some research on yoga today.
Is there a class near you?
Do you have a friend who might like to start with you?
Is there a trial class you could attend this week?

While a physical exercise, yoga is a wonderful tool to deal with stress and learn
to use breathing to relax the body and centre yourself. There are three main
types of yoga: ashtanga, vinyasa and hatha. Hatha is a general term covering
many different types of yoga. It is slow and gentle, a good introduction for
beginners. Vinyasa is more vigorous and based on a series of postures called
sun salutations. Ashtanga is a fast-paced, intense form of yoga. It is a set series
of poses always practised in the same order. It is very physically demanding.

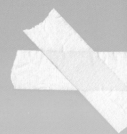

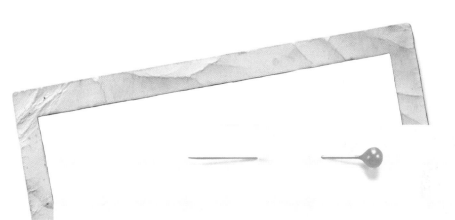

Reducing your 'mum stress'

Get on the computer today and make a reward or star chart for each of your children.
Explain it to them and give them a star for each positive thing they do, for not fighting and for following house rules.

Star charts are a great way to reward children for doing the right thing.
They are also a great way to reduce your stress and they give your children motivation to do the right thing and make your life easier!

Spring in your step

It's a beautiful spring day.
Get outside.
Pack up the dog, the kids or just the water bottle and go for a long walk.
Look around.

Spring is a beautiful time to soak up the energy of new life and enhance your wellbeing.

Ease those aching legs

It's so annoying when you finally get into bed ready for a good night's sleep and your legs just won't stop aching.
Try these ideas to ease the ache:

- Wear supportive shoes throughout the day and elevate your feet when you sit down at night. If they are swollen, lie down and raise them higher than your heart.
- Have a warm bath or foot soak before bed. Add some lavender or ylang ylang essential oil.
- Boost the magnesium in your diet by eating more leafy green vegetables, nuts, seeds, apples, bananas or broccoli.
- Massage your calves using a relaxation oil blend. With long, smooth strokes work along the lines of the aching muscles, from your ankle up to your knee.

Aching legs are a common symptom that can stop us from getting a good night's sleep. Keep a relaxation essential oil blend on your bedside table so you can give yourself an effective leg massage without even having to get out of bed. You will drift off to sleep before you know it.

The eyes have it

If you sit and look at a computer screen for many hours a day, stop and do these exercises today to give your eyes some rest and rejuvenation.

- Moving pencil: Find a coloured pencil and slowly move it to and from the eye while continually focusing on it.
- Palming: Put the palm of your hand over one eye and look around with the other. Look at objects far and near. Change hands to exercise the other eye.
- Magic pencil: Pretend your nose is a pencil. Trace around objects in the room with your 'pencil'.

Continual use of a computer challenges our eyes. Between 50 and 90 per cent of computer workers report some symptoms of computer vision syndrome (CVS). Aside from glare, one of the major problems is that your eye has the same focal point for a long period of time. Simple eye exercises such as those above help to change your eye's focal point and so reduce the chance of them 'locking up' and your eyes becoming tired.

Walking with tins

When you go for a walk today or even as you walk around the house doing your daily chores, carry some small weights with you.
If you don't have small hand weights, use some full food tins.

Small weights increase your load when you exercise and work more muscle groups. This makes your exercise more effective. It means that you burn more calories and tone more muscles. Toned muscles burn more calories than untoned ones.

Clear head space

Clean out your junk drawer today.

We all have a drawer full of junk and every time we open it, we think 'I must clean that out'. It takes up that little bit of our head space. Clean it out today. You will feel a little better for it and it will help clear that cluttered head space.

Nose blaster

Feeling a little blocked in the sinus area?
While the blooming flowers are lovely, their pollens can
wreak havoc with our noses.
Use this sinus flush to clear them out.
Combine 50 grams (1¾ ounces) fresh lemon juice,
1 teaspoon horseradish,
1 crushed garlic clove and 1 tablespoon honey, then strain.
Build up to taking 1 teaspoon four times a day.

Blocked sinuses are the perfect place for bacteria to breed and infection to
take hold. This combination will clear your sinuses but may knock your socks off,
so try a small amount first and build up to the full dose.

File your bills

File your bills today.

It's a horrible, boring job but you will feel good when it's done and it will help to organise your mind and so clear your head. All of these little jobs reduce our stress and so they are worth the time.

Nail secrets

Our nails are another of the body's ways to communicate with us about our health.
Flat spoon-shaped nails can indicate low vitamin B12.
Nails that chip, crack, peel or break easily can be a sign that you need a mineral boost.
Those vertical or horizontal ridges can indicate that your digestion and absorption needs a tune-up.
Many white spots may be an indication of a mineral deficiency or a result of injury.

Understanding the ways your body communicates with you is an excellent way to be proactive with your health. Your nails, hair, tongue and face are used in many alternative medicine systems to indicate of what is going on inside the body. Study your nails to understand what is normal for you, and check them for any changes.

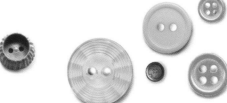

Stretch it

Stretch.
Stand up and reach as high as you can.
Move around so you stretch each and every muscle.
Remember your calves, hamstrings, arms, neck and even the soles of your feet.
Breathe in and out as you stretch.

All animals love to have a stretch, but humans seem to forget to do it. It feels wonderful to stretch everything and get it moving.
Get into the habit.

Tai chi

Go online today and do some research on tai chi.

Watch one of the many free instructional videos and try a simple exercise.

Find out where a class is in your area.

Talk to the teacher and ask about their experience.

Commit to three lessons before you decide if you will make it part of your regular routine.

The 'chi' in tai chi means energy. This slow, soft and graceful martial art is designed to promote the healthy flow of energy through the body, is designed to promote the healthy flow of energy through the body, removing blockages and restoring balance. Tai chi is an exercise in balance, coordination, physical control and breathing. It evolved from ancient Chinese philosophies including Confucianism and Taoism, and is practised by millions worldwide. Just fifteen minutes a day will help to connect all parts of you—body, mind and spirit.

Silky smooth hands

Give your hands a treat today.
Mix together ½ tablespoon fresh lemon juice
and 1 tablespoon sugar.
Now give your hands a good scrub with the mixture.
Rinse off and moisturise.

People always cringe when I ask them to show me their hands in my clinic.
Few people like to show them off. This scrub takes five minutes and will give your
hands a real lift.

Naughty but nice

Have some racy sex today.
Lights on, lights off, doesn't matter.

Sex is a huge part of an intimate relationship. It can make us feel loved, wanted, young and alive. Life can get in the way of sex and make it a low priority. Give it top priority today and make it racy!

The rainbow diet

Eat four pieces of different coloured fruits or vegetables today!
The different colours of fruits and vegetables hint at what each food offers you.

Red and purple foods (strawberries, grapes, currants, blueberries) are rich in vitamin C and give your immune system a boost.
Green foods (apples, broccoli, spinach) are filled with vitamins A, C, E and magnesium and iron. They are fantastic for a healthy heart, nervous system and muscles.
Orange and yellow foods (oranges, lemons, pumpkin, carrots) are rich in vitamin A, which is a strong antioxidant and boosts your skin and teeth.

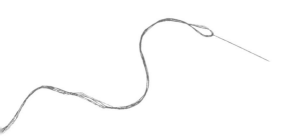

Feed your hair

Whisk up 2 raw eggs, work them through your hair, and leave to dry. Using cool water, rinse out then shampoo your hair. Then rinse with water and a small amount of vinegar for smooth, moisturised hair.

There's nothing quite like a bad hair day. You start the day on the back foot. Taking time to nourish and look after your hair can help you to feel good about who you are when you look in the mirror each morning.

It's all about you

Take this one day to think of yourself first.
It's all about you.
You deserve it.

Every now and then you need to treat yourself like a princess. If you treat yourself well, you will let others treat you well too, and you will begin to believe that you really do deserve it.

Summer

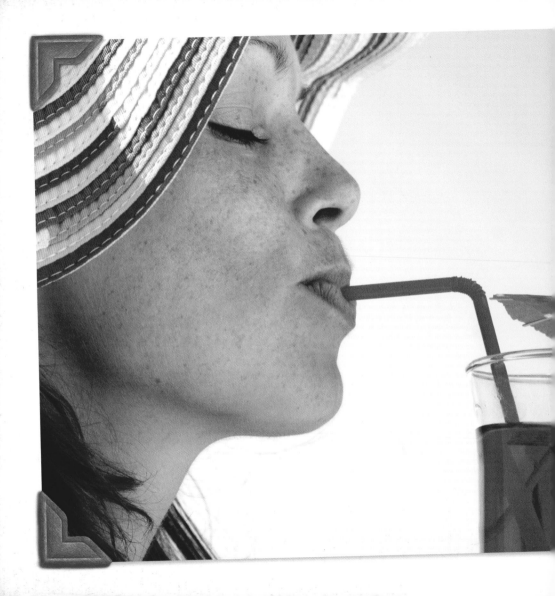

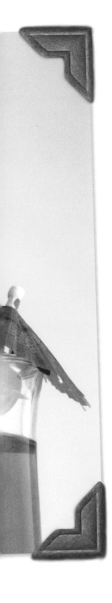

The summer sun fills our world with warm, vibrant light and entices us outside to enjoy the world's natural wonders.

The season is filled with a happy energy and carefree childhood memories. Drinking homemade lemonade under a shady tree, listening to the familiar hum of cicadas, feeling the tightness of salty ocean water as it dries on your skin, smelling freshly cut grass as the mowers do their work.

With windows open, the fresh summer breeze and warmth of the sun fill our homes and lighten our hearts with their healing energy.

Summer diet

The sun has once again returned to the skies and we are all thawed out from the chills of winter.
Wear bright, colourful clothes and get up earlier to go for a walk to soak up the beautiful, healing early morning sunshine.
Change to your summer diet today.
This means introducing lots of cooling, colourful foods back into your diet.
Salads, juices and raw foods all invite the energy of summer back into our bodies and keep us cool.

The energy of summer is lighter than spring, but it can also be hot and overbearing. Eating lots of cool seasonal foods, such as cucumber, sprouts, watermelon, limes, lemon, celery and lettuce, gives us the energy of summer and helps us to keep cool on the inside.

Summer solstice

Look up on the internet the date of this year's summer solstice.
Mark it in your diary.
Plan a small ceremony to celebrate the solstice and be thankful for the gift of another summer.

Shakespeare's *A Midsummer Night's Dream* is set during the summer solstice as it is a magical time of year. It marks the very middle of summer, the longest day of the year, and is a wonderful day to celebrate and be grateful for the beauty, warmth and energy that summer brings.

Indulge yourself

Have a gelato today
and feel like you deserve it.
Enjoy every little bite.

It is important to watch what we eat, but it is also
important to enjoy an occasional treat without guilt or
regret. In moderation, treats are a wonderful part of life.
Allow yourself to enjoy them.

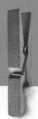

Neck rub

Learn this simple neck rub today
and you will have an instant mobile pick-me-up.
Sit with your back straight, shoulders relaxed,
and take a deep breath.
With or without oil, using the tips of your fingers, run from the
base of your neck right up to the base of your skull.
Start just behind your ears and work around towards the nape
of your neck until your hands meet in the middle of your neck.
Repeat.
Now move your fingers to the base of your skull just behind
your ears. Using small circles, move along the base of the
skull until your fingers meet in the middle. Allow your neck
and shoulders to relax. Repeat.

When our neck muscles get sore, tight or achy, we can suffer from headaches,
tiredness or just a feeling of being out of balance. Doing this simple, gentle neck
rub can help to loosen the muscles and relax the area. If you have any neck injuries
or chronic problems, ensure you see your health professional before you self-treat.

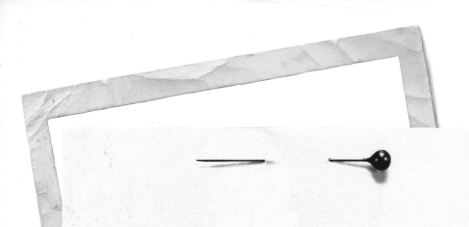

Hair lift

Give your hair a lift today with a natural rinse.
Wash and condition as normal, then do a final rinse with
beer or natural yoghurt. Work the beer or yoghurt through
the hair and comb before rinsing out with water.

These quick and natural rinses will feed your hair and add shine and lustre,
leaving it feeling soft and bouncy.

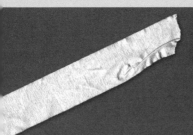

Sweet little stevia

Plan a trip to the garden centre or health food shop on the weekend.
Buy a stevia plant, powder or liquid extract.
Use it in place of sugar in your cooking, baking and drinks.
Experiment to get the sweetness right for you.

Stevia is a sweet plant. It is sweeter than sugar but has no calories and actually works in the opposite way to sugar in the body. It helps to balance blood sugars, does not feed yeasts and other bacteria as sugar does and contains a whole host of beneficial minerals. It's worth a try.

The scent of summer

Celebrate the warmest of seasons with an essential oil blend filled with summer's fresh smells. Blend together 3 drops each of lemongrass, lime and grapefruit for a fresh, citrusy summer blend. Burn in your oil burner.

Blend as you go or make a small bottle of the blend to use throughout the summer. If you have only one or two of the oils, it will work just as well.

Be kind

Do one kind thing for yourself today.

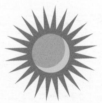

Being kind to yourself is one of life's simple pleasures. It allows you to open yourself to possibilities and reminds you that you are worthwhile and important.

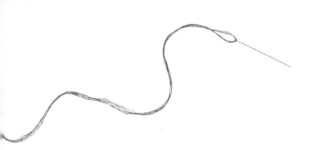

Energise!

Let's give your energy a boost today.
Buy or make a fresh juice using apple, orange and carrot.
Drink it immediately after juicing and enjoy the energy kick
it gives you.

Apples, oranges and carrots are all rich in the vitamins and minerals
we need to make energy. Juicing them is a great way to harness their
goodness and give you a quick burst of energy.

Sexy skin

For smooth and silky skin all over, try this sexy skin scrub today.

Thoroughly mix together 3 teaspoons salt, 2 teaspoons sugar, 2 teaspoons vegetable oil and 2 drops lavender oil.

Jump in the shower and wet yourself thoroughly.

With the water turned off, rub the scrub all over your body, avoiding your face.

Turn the water back on and rinse the scrub off.

It can be hard to peel off the layers we became used to during the cold weather but as the warmer months descend on us, we need to. This sexy skin scrub is a great way to welcome the warmer weather and get your body ready for your summer wardrobe.

Make someone's day

Give a compliment to a woman you don't know.

'We make a living by what we get, but we make a life by what we give.' Winston Churchill.

Deal with it

Make a concerted effort to deal with stress as it
happens today.
Be conscious of your shoulders becoming tight,
your stomach tying itself in knots or your breath
becoming shallow.
Relax your shoulders, take a deep breath,
have a sip of water.
Just being conscious of your stress can dilute its
potency and stop it building up throughout the day.

Everyday stress is often a collection of small triggers that band
together and wreak havoc on our bodies. Often, the most simple act
can short circuit stress and help us become aware of the effects it has
on us before it causes bigger physical and emotional problems.

A handy story

Look at people's hands today to get some clues about their disposition.
Move their hand so that it is open with the thumb out, but still relaxed.
If the four fingers are close together and the thumb is extended ninety degrees without any force, the person has a balanced disposition.
If the angle is less than 90 degrees, they like to abide by conventions and traditions, and may struggle with change.
If the angle is more than 90 degrees, they may not take advice from others well.

The study of the hand and palm is called palmistry and is an ancient art. It has been used throughout the ages to discern a person's character, health and fate. Aristotle (384–322 BCE) found a treatise on palmistry on an altar for the god Hermes. Julius Caesar used it to judge the value of his soldiers.

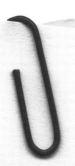

Pick your battles

Give yourself a break today.
Does it really matter if your child is on their Wii, DS,
PSP or computer for a little longer today?
Give yourself a day off from policing the small things.

Giving yourself permission to take a break can help to reduce your
chances of parenting burnout, that combined feeling of being
overwhelmed, frazzled and on the edge of your nerves.

Natural antiseptic

Summer brings with it wonderful weather for running around and being active.
Cuts, bumps, bruises and scrapes are also a part of it. Put some tea tree oil in your natural first aid kit today. It is a wonderful natural antiseptic and antifungal.

Tea tree oil comes from the leaves of the *Melaleuca alterifolia*. In indigenous bush medicine, the melaleuca leaves were crushed and used to heal cuts, burns and infections. The oil of the leaves is antiseptic, antifungal and antibiotic. It is wonderful for use on athlete's foot, dandruff, insect bites, acne, and all manner of cuts and scrapes. You can even add a few drops to some warm water and wipe over home surfaces prone to mould. Always remember to dilute it (1:4 for children), only use it externally, and don't use it if you are pregnant or breastfeeding.

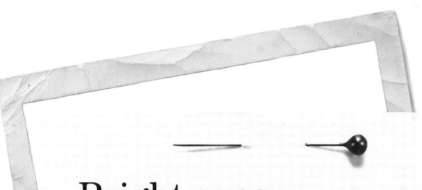

Bright eyes

Give your eyes a boost today.
Feed them with foods rich in vitamins A, C, E and B2.
Pamper them by lying down with a cold tea bag or a slice of cool cucumber on each eye and resting for five minutes.
Have them checked by an optometrist if you're due for a check-up.

Nearly 80 per cent of the information we take into our brains is through our eyes. Taking time to care for them before anything is amiss can pay wonderful dividends. Vitamin deficiencies can cause myriad problems for your eyes so a good diet is vital for their health.

Make a colour statement

Paint your toes with some nail varnish.
Treat yourself to a daring new colour.

Each colour has a different meaning. Red means energy, strength, passion and desire. Pink is all about romance, love and friendship. Orange combines the fire of red and the happiness of yellow. Blue denotes knowledge, depth and integrity, and black is for authority, power and mystery.

The wonders of yoghurt

The superfood for today is natural yoghurt.
Buy it unsweetened and unflavoured.
If you don't like the taste, flavour it yourself with some fresh
fruit such as mashed ripe bananas, mango or strawberries.
Have it for breakfast, a snack or dessert today.

Natural, unflavoured yoghurt is high in a whole host of cancer-fighting
goodies. It is also rich in acidophilus, an essential component for good
digestive health and immunity.

Take the sting from sunburn

No matter how many times we apply the sunscreen,
the summer sun can still burn our skin.
Try these natural soothing alternatives.
Gently bathe sun-burned areas with a soft cloth
dipped in cold tea.
If you have an aloe vera plant in the garden,
cut a leaf off and use the gel to soothe the burn.
Apply some cool sliced cucumber or raw potato to draw
out some of the heat.

If all else fails take a cool bath. Tie some oatmeal into a
sock or stocking and let the water run through it as you
draw the bath. Oats are naturally soothing to the skin
and will help to reduce the heat and itch.

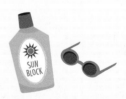

Getting to the heart of it

Think about the health of your heart today.
Not your cholesterol or your circulation but the emotional health of your heart.
In traditional Chinese medicine, the heart is the seat of joy and if the heart is out of balance, we can experience insomnia, crying or even extreme hysteria.
In balance, we experience happiness and joy.
Think about your emotional health and any impediments to joy.
How could these impediments be overcome to allow joy into your life?

In Western culture, the heart is the centre of emotion and where love is felt. Taking the time to think about our feelings and emotional health can have a wonderful effect on our physical health.

Watch the sunset

Watch the sunset this evening. Don't speak, just watch and allow the colours and beauty of it to bring you a sense of peace and wonder.

Even if you only have five minutes to spend watching the sunset, you will still feel the benefit.

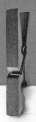

Liquid calories

Are you a sneaky milkshake fan, a smoothie nut or a latte tragic?
Think about your drinks today.
It makes no difference to the taste to have low-fat milk in your
shake or smoothie and will not lessen your enjoyment.
You can re-train your tastebuds to love skim-milk lattes.
Start on your trim drink routine today and stick with it for the next
two weeks to give your tastebuds a chance to adjust.
It will be worth the effort.

Research has found that drinking does not trigger the same satiation or fullness
centre in our brain the same way that food does. This means that if you drink a
high-fat or high-calorie drink, your body doesn't add it to your 'food tally' for the
day and you will be just as hungry at mealtime as you would have been without the
drink. A large full-fat caffe latte contains more calories than a Magnum ice-cream,
so make sure you take juices, milk-based and other potentially calorie-laden drinks
into account if you are watching what you eat.

Love the skin you're in

Give your skin a boost today.
The best way to feed your skin is to drink lots of water, get a good night's sleep and eat foods rich in vitamin E and other antioxidants, such as blueberries, blackberries, strawberries, red grapes, pecans, carrots, tomatoes and broccoli.
Give your skin a gentle scrub with a loofah and soak in a bath with rose or lavender essential oil, sunflower oil and a dash of apple cider vinegar.

Feed, protect, hydrate and clean are the four cornerstones of maintaining lovely, glowing skin. Antioxidants help to protect skin from the pollutants and other nasties in the environment. Giving it a gentle loofah helps to remove the outer layer of dead cells, leaving the new skin cells on the surface.

It's time to talk

Make time to have coffee with a friend today.

Good friends have few expectations of us. They accept us for who we are and support us through the good, the bad and the ugly. Look after your circle of friends and find time for them. It will enrich your life and do wonders for your health and wellbeing.

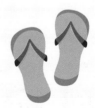

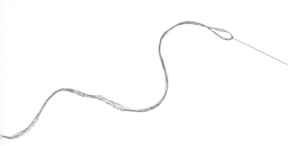

Cool it

Try this cooling summer drink today.
Blend together ½ cup low-fat Greek yoghurt, ½ cup chilled water, 1 teaspoon fresh mint leaves and 2 cups of any summer fruit you have.
Blend until frothy and serve with ice cubes. Add 1 teaspoon of pure maple syrup if you have a sweet tooth.

This lovely summer drink is based on the ayran, a popular Turkish drink, and the lassi, a popular Indian Punjab drink. It is cooling but also has great nutritional benefits. The yoghurt is a source of probiotics ('good bacteria') and calcium, and the mint aids digestion.

Freckle fade

Summertime is when your freckles are really on show. If you want to help them fade, try dabbing on some lemon juice or cucumber and keep out of the sun. Dab on some strong parsley tea or make a mask of ground rosehips and cucumber juice. Apply the mask for fifteen minutes then wash off.

Freckles are like curly hair. Those who don't have them love them. Those who have them can't stand them. There are some commercial products available to help them fade, but using these natural alternatives will help to reduce your chemical exposure.

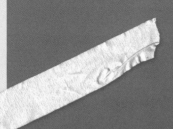

Go with green

Connect with the world today and wear some green.
Light green or dark, it doesn't matter.
It will have the same healing effect on you and those
around you.

In colour therapy, green is considered the master healer. It sits in the
middle of the colour spectrum between the warm and cool ends. It is
the colour of plant energy, chlorophyll, a wonderful tonic and can help
us feel balanced and, green being the most prominent colour in nature,
connected with the world.

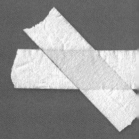

Free to forgive

Forgive someone today.
It may be the person who doesn't hold the door open for you when your hands are full, the guy who steals your car space or someone who has wronged you in the past. Don't waste your energy and get cross.
Let it go and forgive them.
You will be doing yourself a great service.

When we hold grudges or refuse to forgive a person, stranger or family member, we hold that within us. It is a burden we carry, not them. By forgiving them, you will release this from yourself and feel a sense of freedom that enriches the spirit.

Tone and heal

Today let's add another cheap and simple natural remedy to your first aid kit.
This is another tissue salt called Calc Fluor, Elasticity.
It works well for haemorrhoids, varicose veins, cracked skin and strained muscles or ligaments, so it will get a good workout from everyone in the family.
Start dosing, as per the instructions on the label, at the first sign of symptoms.

Cheap, safe and effective, tissue salts are an excellent addition to your first aid kit. The chewable little pills are fast acting and child friendly.

You're having a laugh

Count how many times you laugh today.
Write it down.
Tomorrow, double it.
The next day, double it again.
By the end of the week, your outlook and
wellbeing will have been transformed.

Psychoneuroimmunology is the study of the connection
between our emotional state and our immune system.
Laughter can transform our emotional state, and is a
wonderful tool for clearing negativity, changing perspective
and connecting ourselves with all that really matters in our
lives. We all know the wonderful feeling straight after a big
belly laugh. Get back into the habit.

No more flies

Write this down: Buy a fly swat.

Summertime is fly time. It sounds so simple, but fly sprays and other chemical insect killers are riddled with chemicals that may be harmful to you and your family's health. A fly swat is an old-fashioned, cheap and highly effective way of reducing the chemicals in your house and killing flies. They also give you a good workout!

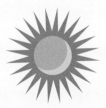

Modern meditation

Most of us say we don't have time to sit and meditate.
Others cannot empty their mind of the 'to do' lists
long enough to relax.
So try some modern meditation or mindfulness.
Have a trial run right now.
What are you sitting on? Does it feel hard or soft?
What noises can you hear around you?
Are there any worries popping into your head?
Let them go.
Can you feel any tension inside your body? Where?
Focus on it, then let it go.
Become aware of your breathing; in and out.
Feel your breath move around your body.

Don't discount meditation until you've tried it a few times to see where
it takes you. Sometimes just letting your inhibitions and perceptions go
and opening up to new possibilities can be liberating.

Glam feet

It's summer and your feet are on show, even in those comfy flip-flops.
Spend a little money on yourself today and get a spa pedicure.
Get your heels buffed, your nails polished and feet massaged.
Your movie star feet will make you feel fabulous!

This is not just about having beautiful feet. This is about feeling like you deserve a little pampering. You're worth it.

Healthy space

A quick lesson in feng shui today.
Feng shui is designed to allow the free flow of positive energy in a space. Here are some very simple feng shui rules you could apply:
Ensure that there is no obstacle or furniture when you enter a room, as it will obstruct the free flow of energy.
A room should be furnished so that you can see anyone who is entering the room.
A mirror on a wall can help with this one.
Your front door and back door should not be aligned or money will come in the front door and straight out the back.

The ancient Chinese system of feng shui uses both the laws of heaven and earth to allow the positive flow of chi (life energy) in a space. It is used to promote health, happiness and prosperity. Records of its use go back thousands of years. In 4000 BCE, dwellings in the ancient Banpo region were placed in line with feng shui beliefs.

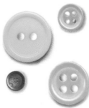

Nude food

Today is all about undressing your food.
No salad dressing, no mayonnaise or sauce,
no sugar or salt.
Try your food whole and undressed.
How long has it been since you tasted its real taste?

We all get into food habits. It may be hot dogs with mustard, relish and sauce or salad with mayonnaise and pepper. Sometimes it is worth having your food undressed for a day to give your body a rest and reconnect with real food. As well as being high in salt, sugar and other preservatives, many condiments hide the real taste of what we are eating.

Move it to lose it

Use the stairs for the rest of the week, don't use the lift.

We all know physical exercise is good for just about everything, but when can we find time to do it? Using the stairs at work, walking to the shop instead of driving, taking the kids to the park instead of sitting at the movies are all ways to include exercise in our current lifestyles. Being conscious of how much we exercise can open up many everyday opportunities to move.

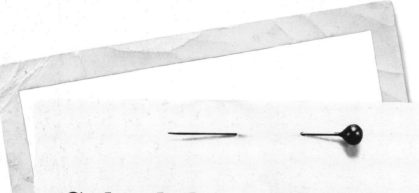

Schedule some fun

Take some time to work out a schedule today.
Could you schedule in some alone time for yourself, an activity or enrichment class, some exercise or play time with the children?

Routines change in different chapters of our lives but they serve a vital role. Time has a way of flying by and a schedule can help you to make the most of your time and enjoy each day. If you have young children, much of your routine is determined by them but you can still find time for yourself here and there if you draw up a schedule. If you live alone, a schedule can help give you structure and purpose each day. It is a wonderful tool if used well.

A Clayton's coffee

Sometimes, we have a tea or coffee just to have a break
from work, or break the monotony of the day,
or to warm us up.
Have you ever seen those 'natural coffee substitutes'
in the coffee aisle of the supermarket?
They taste nothing like coffee, but some of them are
delicious in their own right and are a very good hot
drink to have if you want to cut down your coffee intake.
They are cheap enough to experiment with, so try a few
of them and see if you find one you like.

'Coffee substitutes' are made from grains including chicory and rye, and
are naturally caffeine-free. They are often an acquired taste, so give them
a few tries before you decide if you like them or not. You can have them
with milk, honey or however you like your usual coffee.

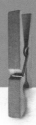

Feel fantastic

Feeling a bit fuzzy around the edges, tired or run down?
Do you have a nagging symptom or just not seem like yourself?
Take ten minutes to do some research today and find a local
natural therapist to get you back on track.
You could read up on naturopathy, polarity therapy, kinesiology,
energetic healing, ayurvedic medicine or any number of natural
therapies—all of which focus on helping to get you bouncing
around again.
Find a therapy you like, then look for a local practitioner.

We often put up with feeling below par because we don't take the time to do
something about it. Always check that therapists are fully qualified and registered
with an authorised registration body. Finding a practitioner you connect with can
make an enormous difference to your health and wellbeing.

Nurture yourself

Every day you give to other people, today give back to yourself. Buy yourself a treat, dress up in something you love, say kind things to yourself, hum a tune, watch some daytime TV, don't do any housework, take a bubble bath.

Nurturing yourself costs little time or money. You just need to make up your mind to do it. You can still go to work, care for the kids, cook dinner, all of the things you usually do, but do a couple of small things within it all to look after yourself and replenish your stores.

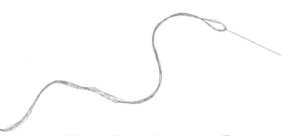

Deliciously smooth

Buy all the ingredients today to have a nutrition-packed
smoothie for breakfast tomorrow.
You will need some frozen mixed berries, natural yoghurt,
skim milk or apple juice and a banana.
Throw it all in the blender in the morning, blend
and drink up.
Make extra for your children or partner; they'll love it.
Your body will thank you for it for the rest of the morning.

A smoothie is a fast and nutritious way to start a summer's day. For a busy
woman, drinking breakfast is faster than eating a bowl of cereal, and for
someone living on their own, most of the ingredients can be frozen so
you won't be throwing out leftovers at the end of the week. Freezing the
bananas then blending them makes for a very creamy smoothie.

Walk away

So you may have been talking about a regular exercise program but have you done anything about it?
Get out and about today.
Go for a walk.
It may only be twenty minutes but get out there.
The hardest part about exercise is movitating yourself to do it, but once you get into the habit it gets much easier and the rewards are huge.

Exercise is beneficial to every aspect of our health and wellbeing. It will keep your weight under control, improve your circulation and fitness, and, best of all, lift your energy, spirits and self-esteem. Summer is a beautiful time to start getting out there, as the days are getting longer and the early morning and evening sun is healing and calming. Once you get serious about your walks, buy a pedometer and build up to 10 000 steps a day. No rush, take it a step at a time.

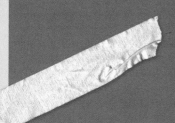

Feeling overwhelmed?

Buy some Cognis Essence today and keep it on hand for those days when you are feeling overwhelmed and that it's all just too much.
We all have those days.
A few drops of Cognis Essence will help to clarify things for you and put you back in the driver's seat.

Cognis essence is part of the Australian Bush Flower Essence range. It's an all-natural product that uses vibrational medicine. It sounds a bit 'out there' but suspend your judgment, give it a try and you will feel the benefits whether you believe in it or not!

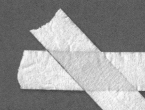

All ears

Listen.
Actively listen today.
When someone is telling you a story, your child is sharing their day or your colleague has some feedback on your work, really listen to what they are saying. Don't think about your reply, think about what they are saying.

Actively listening to people is wonderfully therapeutic for both parties. It invites a deeper sense of connection and understanding, particularly between a parent and child. Children love to be actively listened to and they know when it is happening. Too often we are considering our response before the other person has finished speaking. Really listening to people will open you to some truths and insights that you would otherwise have missed.

Fountain of youth

Start a simple new regime today.
Wear sunscreen on your face
and hands every day.

The sun speeds up the ageing process and the hands
and face are the first place it shows. Wearing a 30+
sunscreen every day will not only help to protect you
from developing melanoma, it will also help to keep you
looking young and beautiful.

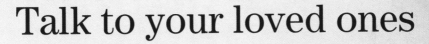

Talk to your loved ones

At the end of the day today, ask your children
or your partner how their day was.
Stop what you are doing and take the time to listen to
their answer.
What were their three favourite things about the day?
The chat may not be a success the first time, but within a
few days, they will begin to enjoy your daily connection
and interest in their world.

Those closest to you love your undivided time and attention. This daily
connection will enrich your relationship with them and help you to further
understand their perspective and what is important to them. It is also a lovely
feeling to reconnect with them at the end of the day.

Lift your lungs

Breathe in and slowly raise your arms above your head, then turn your palms upwards towards the sky, pointing the fingers towards each other.
Rest them on the top of your head.
Breathe out as you straighten your arms towards the sky and press your feet into the ground.
Hold for a second, then breathe in again and move your hands back down to the top of your head.
Repeat five times.

This is a chi kung exercise called 'Supporting the Sky'. Chi kung means 'internal energy exercise' and combines breathing techniques with precise movements and mental concentration to achieve health and wellbeing.

Still waters run deep

Take ten minutes to be still.
Right now.
Clear your mind.
Concentrate on only your breathing.
Just sit there.

It is amazing that we always have this beautiful peace if only we stop for a moment and claim it. This is so simple and yet so effective for recentring ourselves and putting everything into perspective.

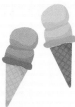

The art of conversation

Are you a good communicator?
Do you listen well?
Do you clearly express your needs and issues?
Do you tell the truth?
Do you complain and natter with your girlfriends but never actually talk to the person concerned?

At work and at home, communication is a key to a happy and harmonious environment, yet few of us are taught how to communicate well. Pay attention to your communication skills today and think about areas where you are great and where you could improve.

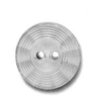

Cool and crisp way to start a summer's day

A perfect summer breakfast will set you up
for a great day today.
Slice up some fresh summer fruits and include some
papaya, strawberries and pineapple. Remember to
include at least part of the chewy core of the pineapple
as it contains lots of enzymes that help your digestion.
Serve with a dollop of natural yoghurt sweetened with
some honey.

The energy of summer is light and bright. It can be harnessed through regularly
eating a range of beautiful summer fruits. Papaya and pineapple are particularly
good as they are rich in papain and bromelain, two excellent digestive enzymes.

Neck stretch

Give your neck a stretch.
Sit down, eyes forward, head straight.
Gently and slowly, move your head to look over your
left shoulder, then your right.
Look up, then down. Repeat.
Now bend your right ear towards your right shoulder.
Repeat on the left side.

Stiff, sore necks are the cause of many headaches. Regular, gentle stretching and
movement can help to keep them supple and well oiled.

Salad friendly

Summer is synonymous with salad.
It is a lovely summer meal.
Make a yummy homemade vinaigrette dressing today to
keep on hand for dressing your salads. In a jar with a lid,
combine 2 teaspoons Dijon mustard with 2 tablespoons
balsamic vinegar and 1 tablespoon extra virgin olive oil.
Cover and shake well.

The only downside of salads is the dressings we put on them. Shop-
bought dressings are often laden with cheap oils, sugar, salt, flavourings,
colourings and bad fats. Making your own dressing is quick and easy, and
ensures you are eating good quality oils and adding something delicious,
but also nutritious, to your diet.

Find your hidden artist

Everybody is creative, you just need to find out where your creativity lies.

Are you a home filmmaker, painter, sculptor, photographer, scrapbooker, writer, chef or dancer?

Think about how and where you could express yourself creatively. Don't worry about others judging you.

You don't have to be Van Gogh, you just have to be you.

The right side of the brain is our creative side. We all have one. It is a wonderful space to play. Most of life uses the logical and rational left side of the brain, which gets the jobs done but gives us little reward. Research shows that people who regularly enjoy or participate in the arts live longer lives. So get creative and live to 100!

Scrub a dub dub

Give your face a gentle scrub today.
Mix together 4 teaspoons yoghurt, 2 teaspoons almond meal, 1 teaspoon oatmeal and 1 teaspoon runny honey.
Gently massage it into the skin.
Rinse off and pat dry.

Scrubs exfoliate the skin, removing all of the dead skin cells and bringing the new, more vital cells to the surface. The result is fresher, softer and younger-looking skin. Lovely!

Tongue tales

Poke your tongue out and look in the mirror.
What does your tongue say about you?
A whitish tongue shows a kapha imbalance and mucus accumulation.
If a tongue is yellowy green, it indicates a pitta imbalance.
A vata imbalance is manifested by a black to brown colouration on the tongue.

Tongue diagnosis is frequently used by ayurvedic and traditional Chinese medicine practitioners as the tongue mirrors the inner workings of the body. Vata, kapha and pitta are the three doshas or constitutional types in ayurvedic medicine. Find a dasha quiz on the internet to see which type best describes you and to give you greater insight into your constitution.

Go team

What about playing a team sport?
It doesn't have to be a serious business,
you can play just for fun.
Netball, basketball, hockey, touch football—get online
and have a look at what is around your area.

We are all told we need regular exercise, but there are a million excuses
as to why we haven't, can't and didn't. Joining a team sport makes
you answerable to eight or more other people, and makes you move
your schedule around so you have the time to exercise. It also helps
you to blow off steam and makes exercise fun as you share it with your
teammates. If you are worried that you won't be good at it, start in a low
division where you feel comfortable.

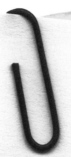

Healthful tea

Make a rosemary tisane today.
Pick or buy 6 sprigs of fresh rosemary.
Place them in a teapot or coffee plunger
and fill with boiling water.
Cover and allow to steep for 5–10 minutes.
Drink it throughout the morning to wake you up,
clear your mind and activate your senses.

Tisanes are infusions of herbs, like herbal teas. They are lovely when made with fresh herbs and apart from tasting delicious, they are a great way to give you a gentle health boost. Rosemary is stimulating, chamomile is relaxing, lemon verbena supports the nervous system and helps digestion, and basil is helpful with colic and other digestive complaints. Avoid rosemary if you are pregnant.

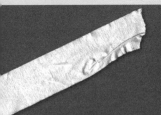

Hair food

Today you are going to feed your hair.
You will need to whisk together 1 egg yolk and 3 teaspoons apple cider vinegar. While whisking, slowly add 4 teaspoons castor oil, 3 teaspoons olive oil and 4 drops rosemary essential oil to the egg and vinegar in a thin stream.
Massage it into your hair and comb through with a wide-toothed comb.
Cover your hair with a shower cap and sit in a warm place for twenty minutes.
Wash out with warm water and then shampoo and condition as normal.

As lovely as it is, the summer sun is unkind to our hair. Give it a feed and lift with this all-natural hair food every fortnight throughout summer. If you don't have any rosemary essential oil, use another of your favourite essential oils or just leave it out.

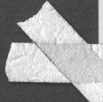

Waterplay

It's summertime.
Time to get in the pool.
Call your local pool today and go along to their
aquarobics session this week.

Water is a wonderful place to exercise. It resists
movement, helping to strengthen your muscles
and give you a good cardio workout but it also
supports you so you don't strain or injure yourself.
It is a lovely exercise for summer and, at most
pools, you only pay for the sessions you go to.

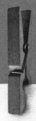

A sunny drink

Try this sunny drink today.
Make a pot of lemon balm or lemon verbena tea
and add a large bunch of fresh mint.
Steep then allow to cool.
Add some ice and sliced lemon.

Not only food can be used to support our health, drinks are a wonderful way
to attune to the rhythms and climate of the season. Using seasonal produce
is a good way to support the body in its tasks. In spring and summer, most of
the seasonal produce is cooling and soothing, helping the body to maintain
its balance in the warmth. This is a beautiful tea for the warmer months.
The lemon balm and lemon verbena are good for the digestive system and
the ice, lemon and mint are cooling and delicious. If you are pregnant or
breastfeeding, omit the mint.

It's not all white

**Don't eat any white food today.
This means white pasta, bread, cakes, biscuits,
anything made with white flour.**

Throughout the manufacturing process, white flour has been stripped of
many of its original nutrients, fibre and goodness. It clogs up our digestive
system and can cause bloating, a feeling of heaviness and a lack of energy.
If you can't bring yourself to say goodbye to it altogether, just take a
periodic break and give your digestive system a rest from it. See how much
better you feel.

Music madness

Remember when you were younger.
If a boy liked you, he would make you a CD (or tape depending on your age!) of the latest and best songs.
Well, let's reminisce.
Make a CD compilation today of your favourite 'get up and dance, sing as loud as you can' songs.
Keep it in the car and whenever you are driving alone, crank it up and sing your heart out.

People in other cars find this endlessly fascinating and you can always see a twinge of envy in their eyes as you play air guitar and make out you are a rock star! For some of us, our time in the car is the only time we have alone so use it to let your hair down and be yourself.

Just desserts

Make some healthy desserts today.
It only takes a few minutes and it is wonderful to
finish dinner and know you have something delicious
and guilt-free in which to indulge afterwards.
Try some fruit juice jelly, low-fat frozen yoghurt or
make some fresh fruit smoothies and freeze them
in iceblock containers.

After dinner is the most dangerous eating time for most people. This is
when the chips, biscuits and chocolates really take centre stage, but it's the
worst time of day to be eating them as you can't burn them off before you
go to bed. Rather than relying solely on your willpower to keep you out of
the fridge, take some action and plan a few healthy and delicious desserts
this week. That way, you are controlling what you are eating and also
having the evening treat you are craving.

Attitude of gratitude

Today the glass if half full.
You are going to be positive
about everything.
Grateful for the good and oblivious
to the bad.

Gratitude and positivity are often learned skills. We need to
make a conscious effort to see things in a positive light and
think of what we do have rather than what we don't. With
practice it becomes second nature and makes everyday life a
whole lot rosier.

Regular checks

Give yourself a breast examination in the shower.
Put a regular time in your diary to remind you of your
monthly check-up.

Get to know your breasts well. Know each bump and curve, so you can readily
detect any changes. Early detection is our best weapon against breast cancer.
It takes less than five minutes a month and could save your life.

Number twos

No-one likes to talk about poo, but today you are going to check the health of your poo. You can do this. The perfect poo is medium brown and neither floats nor sinks. It's like a Mr Whippy ice-cream. How does yours compare? Do your bowels need more fibre? More water? More time to move each day? Think about it.

Naturopaths love to talk about poo, as it tells us so much about the inner workings of the body. A healthy bowel and superb poo are key components of good health.

Wardrobe cleanse

Go through your wardrobe today.
Give away anything that you have not worn in the last two
years, no matter how much you paid for it.

There is such a sense of freedom in cleaning out your wardrobe. It helps you
let go of the past and embrace the present and future. Old clothes are full of
emotions, ranging from guilt, regret, sadness and disappointment to joy, love
and excitement. Keeping the wrong clothes hanging in your wardrobe can make
you feel fat, daggy, old and stuck in the past. Don't be afraid to let them go and
give the emotions and bad memories away with them. Sometimes it can take a
couple of attempts to do a thorough clean-out, so plan a follow-up in a week and
you will feel like a new person.

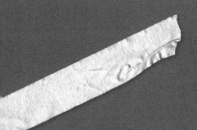

Become a brainiac

Help to reduce brain fog by giving your brain a boost today. Cut some fresh rosemary or basil, make some gingko tea, or have a cup of miso soup.

Rosemary is an excellent stimulant for the brain, aiding mental sharpness and recall. Use fresh rosemary or burn the essential oil. Basil and gingko help the circulation of your blood, to ensure your brain is receiving all of the oxygen and other goodies it needs. As miso is very salty, it has a contracting effect on the body, clearing the mind and increasing your clarity. Buy it fresh or use the conveniently packaged miso soup.

Work less

Don't do any unnecessary work today.
If it can be done tomorrow, leave it for tomorrow.
Give yourself an easy day.
You deserve it.

This is a day to have a mini recharge. You may still have all of your usual
work and home duties, but don't do more than you need to. Let those
batteries charge up. Go on, watch a little daytime TV.

Chocolate-free day

Today is a chocolate-free day.
Yes, you can do it.

If you have read past the heading, then you really
are committed to making some changes! Give
your body a rest from chocolate today.
Find some other activity or non-food comfort
to get you through the day.

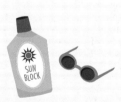

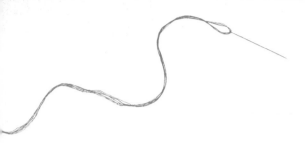

Emotional check-in

In traditional Chinese medicine the spleen is a key organ that is pivotal to our health and wellbeing. The positive emotions attached to the spleen are pensiveness and thoughtfulness. If the spleen energy is blocked, the emotions become worry and obsession and you feel run-down, sluggish and tired.

The season for the spleen is late summer, so now is the time to think about rebalancing the emotions and feelings that are attached to the spleen.

If your 'spleen emotions' are feeling out of balance, try spending less time in your head and more time doing and acting. Go for a run in the sunshine, feel the wind in your hair, laugh, bushwalk, listen to the birds singing, play a game with your children. Move out of your head space and into the physical world to find a balance between thinking, acting and feeling.

One day detox

Your body is your temple.
Make today a mini detox day.
Start with a vegetable juice for breakfast.
No alcohol, wheat or dairy for the day.
Lots of fruit and vegetables.
And 2 litres (3½ pints) of filtered water.

Detoxing allows organs which filter and break down foods, chemicals and toxins to be flushed out. By having only pure foods and drinks for a day, you give your organs time to rest and restore.

Open your mind

Talk to three people at work you have never spoken to before.

It is great to challenge ourselves and move out of our comfort zones. It makes us grow, explore and change our perspective. There may be people in your everyday life who have much to offer you or teach you but need to be invited in. Open your mind.

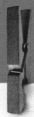

Drink some sunshine

Make or buy a sunshine smoothie today to bring the joy and lightness of summer into your body.
Blend together some ice, cranberry juice, mixed frozen berries and fresh mint.
Serve with a cocktail umbrella.

Eating and drinking the fruits of the season are good ways of moving with nature's and your body's natural rhythms. The berries in this smoothie are rich in vitamin C, bioflavinoids and many other nutrients needed to give you a boost and help you feel sunny.

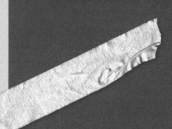

Give yourself a spray

Get a spray tan today.
Go on, bring a little Hollywood into your life.

Spray tans make you look great and when you look into the mirror and like what you see, it does wonders for your self-esteem and wellbeing. Get an organic spray tan done in a salon or do it yourself at home. However you do it, it covers any lumps and bumps and makes you look like a movie star.

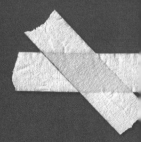

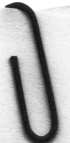

Heel makeover

It's late in summer.
How have your feet fared through these hot months?
Check your heels today.
If they are looking cracked and dry, take time to rub in some almond or vitamin E oil, and use a natural pumice stone in the shower every day to remove the dead skin and get them back to baby smooth.

The lovely open-backed shoes of summer can leave our heels cracked, dry and sore. Taking some regular time to care for them helps to keep our feet looking great and prevent longer term foot problems.

Boost your energy

Green foods and drinks (such as chlorophyll, wheat grass juice or spirulina) are wonderful for boosting your energy, as are wholegrain carbohydrates (none of that white stuff). Increasing your water intake and making sure you eat enough lean protein are also great ways to boost energy production. This means foods like lean meat and legumes.

The body's energy-production cycle is a beautifully complex system that requires many different raw materials to keep it working efficiently. Green foods (rich in B vitamins and minerals), wholegrain carbohydrates (rich in slow-release glucose) and protein (rich in the body's building blocks) all help to keep the cycle turning. Water is the great lubricant.

Storytime

Write a story of a time when you felt truly happy.
Fold it up and keep it in a special place.

Your happy story can be a wonderful way to pick yourself up when you are down. Take it out and read it when you need some sunshine in your life.

Summertime drink

Make a jug of iced tea today.
Choose a herbal citrus variety such as lemon.
Add lots of ice, fresh sliced lemon and a teaspoon of
honey if you like it sweet.
Sip on it throughout the day for an instant pick-me-up.

Iced tea is a lovely summer drink. Making your own is quick, easy,
caffeine-free and gives you a change from water.

Food facial

Give yourself a five-minute facial today.
Mash half an avocado and combine it with a
beaten egg.
Apply the mask to your face and put a slice of
cucumber over each eye.
Lie down for ten minutes and relax before
washing it off.

Don't bother buying an expensive face mask when you can
whip this up in the kitchen. It feeds your skin and leaves it
feeling lovely, soft and chemical-free.

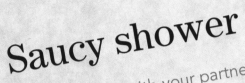

Saucy shower

Have a shower with your partner today.

Bit saucy, isn't it, but fun!
Go on, drop those inhibitions.
Your partner will love it.

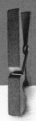

Wonder potion

This wonder potion awaits you today.
Buy some Bach's Rescue Remedy spray, drops or
pastilles from your health food store or chemist, and use
it freely to bring peace and calm to your life, home and
family.

Bach Flower Remedies are made from the energy of flowers and have
been used to great effect since they were discovered by Dr Edward
Bach in the 1930s. Four drops (or sprays) of Rescue Remedy under the
tongue brings an immediate sense of calm and peace. It's great for your
handbag, office desk or kitchen drawer.

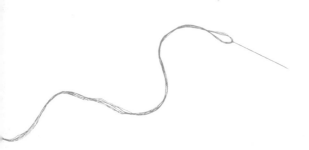

Enrol in a course

Pick up a brochure for a community college today.
They are at local libraries and also online.
Courses are cheap, fun and let you play and learn in areas
that you may have never considered.
It's a great way to broaden your mind and social network.

Short courses are excellent for awakening sides of yourself that may
have, to date, been dormant. They can be serious, fun or open up the
possibility of a new vocation. They break the routine and bring some
fun and excitement into your life.

A cleansing day

Eat lots of liver-loving foods today—carrot, beetroot, alfalfa sprouts, lecithin and green leafy vegetables. Bitter greens such as kale, rocket and endive are great too.
Drink at least 2 litres (3½ pints) of filtered water, and try some dandelion tea.

With all the chemical exposure and the high level of processed foods in our diet, our liver has an enormous workload. Poor sleep, irritability, sluggishness, low mood, tiredness and poor digestion can all be symptoms of a poorly functioning liver, so feed it well and give it a rest and you will reap the benefits. This one-day liver-loving exercise is just a taste of a liver cleanse which would usually last from one to six weeks.

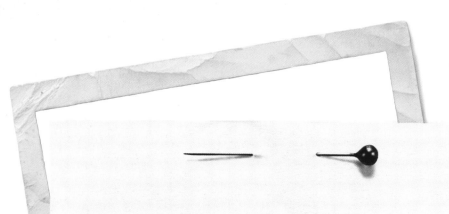

Clean lunch

Have a salad for lunch today, no dressing.

Food is not just for enjoyment. It is also to nourish our body and fuel our mind. At least a couple of days a week, think about your body with your food choices instead of your tastebuds. It is even easier to do this in the warmer months of summer, as salads and light meals are what most of us crave. A clean salad a couple of times a week will fuel you well and give your body a boost of goodies.

Autumn

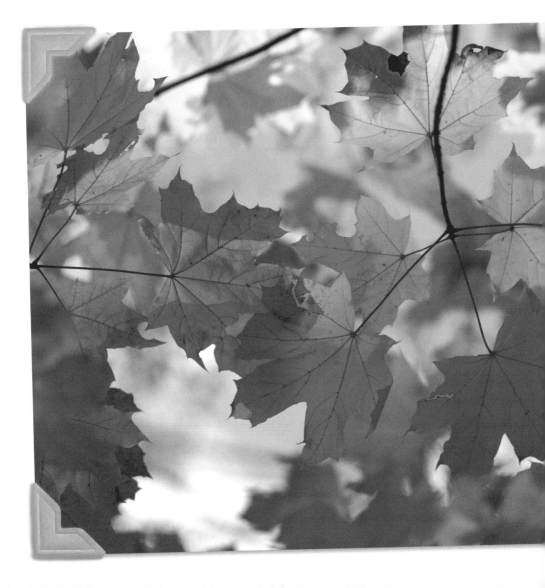

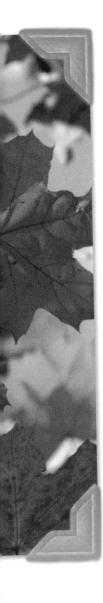

The new energy of spring and the heat of summer have faded as we now roll into autumn, nature's season of harvest. The seeds are ready to be lifted by the autumn winds and carried to fertile soil where they'll wait for the spring.

Autumn is a season of transition for all of nature. We see the leaves change to their autumn hues of red, yellow and ochre before they fall. It's a beautiful time of year—look upon the changing leaves, listen to their crunch under your feet, smell the cool freshness of the coming winter.

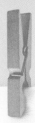

Autumn diet

The harvest has begun and the leaves are beginning to fall. Our energy begins to move inwards and downwards in preparation for winter. It's time to change to a nurturing autumn diet today. No more cold salads or raw foods. Focus on warm well-cooked foods and start using lots of chilli, curry, garlic, cinnamon and ginger in your cooking.

Autumn is here, signalling that winter is on its way. Now is the time to fortify and nurture ourselves and our family from the cold and begin to warm our insides. Garlic, chilli, curry, ginger and cinnamon are all warming and contain phytonutrients which help to boost our immune system and fight against colds and flus. Other great autumn foods include apples, pears, sweet potato, zucchini, carrots, figs, leeks, eggs, green beans, oranges and pumpkin.

Wonder soup

Make a big pot of vegetable soup for dinner tonight.
Use as many different coloured vegetables as you can.
Focus on the wonder vegetables including broccoli,
cauliflower, collard greens, brussel sprouts, kohlrabi,
cabbage, bok choy, komatsuna, radish and rutabaga.
Some of these you may not know. Pick one you don't
know from your fruit and vegetable shop, and add it
to your soup.

These wonder vegetables are all called cruciferous vegetables and have
a distinct mustardy taste. Their health benefits are amazing as they are
high in vitamin C, selenium, soluble fibre and fantastic phytonutrients
such as indole-3-carbinole, which has strong anti-cancer properties.

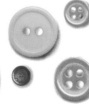

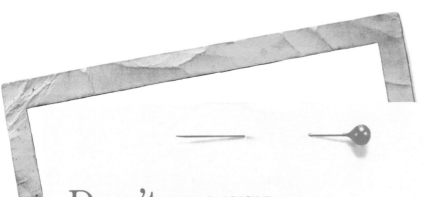

Don't worry

'Worry gives a small thing a big shadow.'
Swedish proverb.
Make a list of all the little things that are worrying you.
Keep the worries on the list and out of your mind. Keep the
list with you and whenever a worry pops into your mind,
write it on the list and leave it there.

Worry serves no positive purpose in your life but can be a hard habit to break.
Writing down worries can help to unclutter your mind and free you to think
about other positive, productive things.

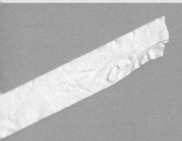

Autumn equinox

Look up on the internet the date of this year's autumn equinox.
Mark it in your diary.
Plan a small ceremony to welcome the equinox as it is the first true day of autumn.

For thousands of years humans have followed the movements of the planets and the ebb and flow of the seasons, the rhythms of the Earth. Reconnecting to these rhythms connects us to our spirit and our higher sense of being. The seasons change according to the movement of the Earth and sun, not the calendar. For this reason, celebrate the equinox and welcome autumn for another year.

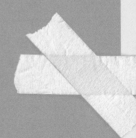

A foot warmer

Keep your feet warm in the cooler months.
Add a handful of fresh rosemary to some almond or
vegetable oil and seal in a glass jar.
Stand it on a light-filled window sill for fifteen days.
Remove the rosemary and replace it with a fresh bunch for
another 15 days.
Strain and store it in a dark glass jar.
Use it in the mornings or evenings to massage your feet.

The rosemary will help to promote circulation and keep your feet lovely and
warm. The massage will help you to relax and keep you connected to your
physical self and your own needs. Your rosemary oil is also an excellent hair
tonic for dandruff or thinning hair. Just rub it directly onto the scalp.

Count your blessings

Tell your partner six things you love about them.
Expect nothing in return.

This will remind you why you fell in love with
your partner and remind them that, beyond
the functional everyday, they are appreciated
and loved.

Hand therapy

While you are in the kitchen today, give your hands some therapy.
Pour a teaspoon of olive oil into them and gently rub it in, getting it into all the little nooks and cracked crannies.
Don't forget your cuticles to keep them nice and soft.
If you have time, wrap them in a warm tea towel for five minutes to allow the oil time to soak in well.

The winds of autumn are very drying to the skin, especially the hands. If you have children, you would also be continually washing your hands, which further dries them. Try using an all-natural soap, such as oatmeal, to reduce the dryness. If your hands are particularly rough and chapped, rub the yellow skin side of a lemon on them to release the natural oils and soften them.

Autumnal oils

Buy or make an autumn blend of essential oils today to fill your home with the heady smells of this harvest season. Blend 3 drops each of juniper, lemon, rosemary and lemongrass essential oils and burn in your oil burner.

Blend as you go or make a small bottle of the blend to use throughout the autumn. If you have only one or two of the oils, it will work just as well.

Assaulting your heart

Become the salt police for a day.
Look at the salt on the nutrition panel of everything
you eat during the day.
Add it up.
How much salt did you consume today?

Processed food manufacturers love salt and so do many of us. Unfortunately, our bodies do not. Salt may taste delicious, but it has a huge long-term effect on our bodies. It effects the way our kidneys work and so also has an impact on our heart. We need some sodium in our diet, but not in the quantities most of us eat. Becoming more vigilant about the amount of salt you eat can really have a positive effect on your heart and kidneys. As a rule of thumb, only eat foods that have less than 120 milligrams (¼ ounce) of salt per 100 grams (3½ ounces) of food. With this gauge in mind, you will be shocked by how high in salt some of your regular foods are.

Sleep insurance

Keep a bottle of an essential oil sleep blend
next to your bed.
Chamomile and lavender blend together well
to encourage sleep.
This evening, rub a small amount into your temples and
on the inside of your wrists before you hop into bed.
The oils will work to soothe your mind and remind your
body to relax and allow sleep to come.

During sleep, the body repairs, renews and re-energises. But there are
times in life when getting a good night's sleep is challenging; you need to
remind your body that it is time to relax and let the day go. Essential oils
are an excellent trigger for the mind to surrender control and ease into a
relaxed sleep.

Smudge stick for autumn

Freshen the air, warm the atmosphere and clear unpleasant smells and energies from your home with this twice-a-year smudge stick.
Traditionally, sage and sweetgrass are used but a bunch of mixed fresh woody herbs such as thyme, lavender or rosemary will work just as well. Tie the bunch together with some pure cotton string and leave in a warm, dry place for a few weeks. When the bunch is dry, carefully light it.
The herbs will slowly begin to smoulder and smoke.
Gently wave the smudge stick around the room. Allow the smoke to transform the air. Once the smell of the herbs has filled the room, extinguish the smudge stick.

As we learned in spring, smudging is a powerful cleansing technique from the Native North American tradition. Always keep a close eye on your smudge stick to ensure that the herbs only smoulder with no flame. To extinguish the smudge stick, dip it into sand and then trim the burnt ends.

Brain box

It's time to give your brain a workout today. Sit down and do a crossword, some Sudoku or another type of puzzle.

Our brain is like a big muscle. The more it works out, the stronger and faster it gets. Giving yours a regular workout will help to improve your mental agility and also give you some quiet time to yourself.

Headache

Before you pop a pill today, try some natural remedies to ease a tension headache.

- Place a small amount of lavender essential oil on the tips of your index fingers and, using small circular movements, gently rub it into your temples. Close your eyes and allow the lavender to do its work.
- Have a warm cup of tea with a small amount of honey. Chamomile tea is excellent for helping you to relax.
- Buy a migraine stick from the health food shop or pharmacy. It is a small stick filled with a combination of herbs. Rub it on your temples and it will help to ease your headache.
- Relax. Simple but highly effective. Go to a quiet place, sit or lie down and let yourself relax, if only for just five minutes. Then write a list of the things you need to do today, in order of priority. And don't forget to ask for help if you need it.

These natural pain relievers take more time than popping a pill, but they are kinder to your body and address the cause of the problem rather than band-aiding it. You may be frantically busy, but taking five minutes to get rid of your headache will be a good investment and make you much more productive for the rest of the day.

Fascia lift

Put a tennis ball under your desk
or next to the couch today.
When you are sitting, take off your shoes and roll
the ball backwards and forwards along the length
of your foot for a few minutes.
Now do the same for the other foot.
Continue to do this throughout the day whenever
you are sitting down.

The plantar fascia supports the arch of the foot. It can get very tight
and sore. The tennis ball roll helps to massage, relax and release
the ligament.

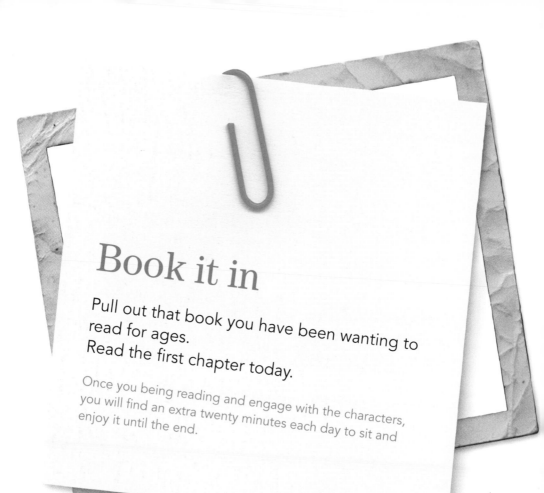

Book it in

Pull out that book you have been wanting to read for ages.
Read the first chapter today.

Once you being reading and engage with the characters, you will find an extra twenty minutes each day to sit and enjoy it until the end.

Crusty skin no more

The winds of autumn can bring with them dry, cracked skin. Try this steam inhalation to rebalance your skin and restore its oils and suppleness.
Combine 4 drops chamomile essential oil, 6 drops orange essential oil, 5 drops geranium essential oil and 3 tablespoons vegetable oil in a glass jar. Shake well.
Use 1 teaspoon of the blend each time you steam your face.

For a steam inhalation, tie your hair back and wash your face. Carefully pour 1 litre (1¾ pints) of boiling water into a bowl or saucepan on a heatproof non-slip mat on a table. Add your essential oil blend, put your face 20–30 centimetres (8–8½ inches) away from the water, cover your head with a towel or large cloth, breathe deeply and relax. Stay there for about ten minutes, then wash your face clean with tepid water. This inhalation will help to feed your skin while also giving you some time to sit and relax. It can also help to keep your sinuses clean and clear.

Just imagine

Is there something you have to do today that you are not looking forward to?
Use the power of your imagination to help manage the anxiety, tension or pain it may be causing.
Close your eyes.
Imagine somewhere you feel safe, happy and secure.
How does it smell, look, feel? What can you hear?
Who is there with you?
What feeling does it give you?
Stay there for a few minutes and allow the tension or pain to leave your body.

Creative visualisation allows you to change your thoughts, moods and behaviour by using only your imagination. At any time, you can close your eyes and take yourself back to your safe haven, once again experiencing the positive feelings and sensations it brings you.

A life line

Have a look at your life line.
It is the deep arc found on the hand that swings
around the thumb on each hand. It can tell you a great
deal about a person. Look at your friends'
and colleagues' hands today and study their lifeline.
A person who does not have a passion for life
often has a life line that runs close to the thumb.
A passionate person who lives life to the maximum
often has a life line that is curved.
People who have delicate health
often have a chained life line.
A person with a heart for travel
often has a life line that swings outwards.

Most people think that, in palmistry, the life line indicates how long you will
live. This is not the case. The life line is an indicator of the amount of vitality,
strength and energy you have for life and quality of the life you live.

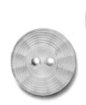

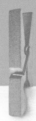

Spot on

If you are having trouble with your skin during the changeable autumn weather, try some of the tissue salt Calc Sulph Blood Cleanser today.
It's a fantastic remedy for spots, pimples, skin disorders and any slow-healing wounds.
Start dosing, as per the instructions on the label, at the first sign of symptoms.

Tissue salts are a homeopathically prepared mini dose of the body's essential minerals. Each tissue salt is composed of a single or combination of minerals which target specific symptoms or complaints. The salts work by restoring the natural balance of the body and ensuring any mineral imbalances are corrected. Always consult your healthcare professional if symptoms persist.

Connect online

If you are not already on Facebook, Twitter or any other social media site, sign up today.

It only takes a minute to sign up and will reconnect you with some of the highlights of your past. You can choose who you do and don't want to connect with. It is a great way to rekindle old friendships and perhaps even old flames.

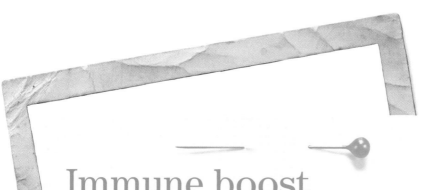

Immune boost

Give your immune system a boost today through these simple steps.

Eat foods rich in vitamins A, C, E and zinc such as citrus fruits, strawberries, carrots, broccoli, eggs, sunflower seeds, corn, wheatgerm, pepitas, oysters, whole grains and cashews.

Try this immune-booster smoothie: $^2/_3$ cup combined apple and blackcurrant juice, ½ cup mixed frozen berries, 1 banana, 1 tablespoon wheatgerm and 1 tablespoon linseed oil.

Deal with stress as it happens. Take a minute to chill out with some breathing or meditation.

Don't have lunch at your desk. Walk somewhere peaceful, sit down and rest to recharge your batteries.

To function well, our immune system needs relief from stress, sound rest to recharge, and abundant raw materials from our diet.

Out of your comfort zone

Try a new food today.
Something you have never tried before.
It may be a legume (such as chick peas) in a salad or curry, a bowl of miso soup, an unusual vegetable or even some tofu.
Try something new and expand your dietary horizons.
You may be surprised and like it.

Trying something new gets you out of dietary ruts and habits. Just adding one new food will help to increase the variety in your diet and so boost the nutrients you offer your body.

A stitch in time

A cold can often be stopped in its tracks
if you recognise and treat it early.
Look after yourself today.
You may have to go to work, but take some fresh lemon and
Manuka honey with you, a wheat bag and a bottle of Breath
Easy or eucalyptus oil on a handkerchief.
Sip warm lemon and honey tea throughout the day, place a
warm wheat bag on your chair so that it covers your kidney
area, and keep the eucalyptus hanky close by so that you
can smell it as you work.

Manuka honey is a specially prepared honey available from most health food
shops. Its therapeutic properties have been widely researched. The honey
contains a phytochemical called UMF, which is strongly antibacterial and
so an excellent tool to ward off a cold or flu.

A shiatsu charge

This shiatsu exercise incorporates the elements of deep breathing, meditation, sound therapy and acupressure.
Sit quietly on the floor, on a cushion or mat, and place one hand on top of the other over the navel.
Breathe deeply, listening to your breath.
Focus on the area about 3½ centimetres (1½ inches) below your navel.
In shiatsu, this point is 'ki-kai' or 'ocean of energy'.
As you continue to breathe deeply and slowly, hum a tune as you breathe out.
After ten breaths, lean forward onto your hands as you breathe out.
Next breathe in, gently straighten your spine and return to your original sitting position. Repeat five times.

This is a very simple shiatsu exercise designed to relax, centre and connect to your 'ocean of energy'. Shiatsu, or finger therapy massage, is a Japanese form of bodywork. It is based on the philosophy that illness and disease result from imbalances in the natural flow of chi (life energy) through the body.

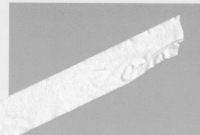

Cheap trick

Buy a bottle of apple cider vinegar today.
From tomorrow morning, begin to take a teaspoon
or two of it each morning in a glass of water.
That's it!

Taking apple cider vinegar sounds like an old folk tale. How can
something so cheap and modest-looking be so wonderful for your
health? Try it and you will see for yourself. It helps to cleanse your
insides, improves digestion and gives you a glow of health. For a
small outlay, it's worth a try.

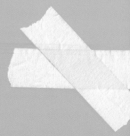

No time like the present

Is there something you have always
wanted to do?
Learn a foreign language, join a choir, play
the bongos or dance the rumba.
Take positive steps and do something
about it today.

I wonder why we put so many things off and then something
terrible happens that threatens our life, livelihood or health
and we decide to adopt a *carpe diem* ('seize the day')
attitude and do all of the things we have been putting off.
Don't wait for that life-changing experience, do it now.

Breathe easy

Autumn is the season for the lungs and so now is a great
time to attend to any issues in that area.
On a physical level, do you have a cough or any
congestion you need to clear?
On a spiritual level, traditional Chinese medicine tells us
that the lungs are the seat of grief and sadness, so dealing
with any unresolved feelings can help to clear the lungs
and keep your chi (life energy) flowing freely through them.

Unresolved feelings do not just go away. They are stored in the body waiting
to be expressed. They will express themselves spiritually, mentally or physically.
Unfortunately for those of us who like to 'sweep things under the carpet',
physical signs of our feelings can show in the form of illness.

Foot rub

Place a towel near the heater for a few minutes
until it is warm.
Then, remove it from the heat
and wrap your feet in it until they are toasty.
Taking one foot out at a time,
massage your feet all over.
If you are feeling tense, take extra time massaging
between the big toe and the second toe to
release the jaw area, a place where many of us
store tension.

The ancient Egyptian, Chinese and Native American Indian cultures
all used a form of reflexology for healing. Reflexology is an energetic
healing therapy. Each organ and part of the body has a corresponding
or reflex area on the foot, hand and ear. In reflexology, pressure is
applied to specific areas on the foot, increasing chi or life energy to
the area and stimulating the body's own healing mechanisms.

Music for harmony

Go online today and download some free meditation music.
Play it while you work to maintain a peaceful and calm environment.

There are some wonderful sites legally offering meditation music for free. There are many different styles of meditation music, so download a few samples to find the style you like. It creates a peaceful, harmonious atmosphere.

Blue to cure the blues

If you are feeling a little hotheaded, stressed or angry today, look out for some blue to soothe you. Taking some time to look at the sky is a wonderful way to bring some blue into your life, as is cuddling up to someone in a blue jumper.

In colour therapy, blue opposes the fiery red and so is cooling and soothing. It can help to calm a fractious nervous system and make us feel more tranquil. It has a calming vibration and can help us feel safe and at peace.

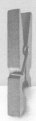

Non-food comfort

What do you do when you feel stressed, anxious, upset or
disappointed? Do you reach for your favourite comfort food?
Think about the times you are most likely to reach for the chocolate,
pudding, cake, biscuits or whatever is your favourite comfort food.
What other non-food comfort could you seek to give you that
pick-up you crave?
Is there a favourite piece of music you could put on, some
breathing exercises, a warm bath you could soak in?
Work out what your non-food comforts are and try to slot them in
when you are next feeling challenged.

Too often we reach for food when we are looking for comfort. It is more about the
comfort than the food. The problem with comfort food is that the good feeling it
temporarily gives us is often replaced by guilt soon after eating it, which just makes
the whole problem worse. Non-food comforts are a great way to break the cycle.

Stress less

Write down the five things which stress you the most.
Now answer these questions.
Can you remove any of them, reduce your interaction
with any of them, change the way you manage them?
If the answer is no to all three questions, develop a quick
and mobile de-stressing technique you can use when you
are stressed by one of them.

Stress can creep up on us. Small thing after small thing start to make our
blood boil and before we know it our blood pressure is through the roof
and we are snappy and irritated. Finding easy things you can do to deal
with stress in the moment will improve your health and wellbeing. It may
be a simple breathing technique, closing your eyes and going to your
special place, listening to some music or going for a quick walk. Work
out what works for you and use it daily to nip your stress in the bud.

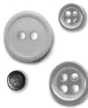

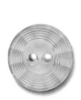

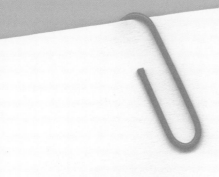

Check-up

You may get your car serviced regularly but when was the last time you had a check-up with your GP?

A good old physical.

If it has been more than a year, give your doc a call and book in. Get a full blood count, check out your liver function, your blood pressure and your cholesterol.

Tell them about any nagging or new symptoms you have and review any medication you are on.

Time goes by so quickly that a year can fly by before we know it. It is great practice to have a wellness check-up with your GP and also your natural health practitioner at least once a year just to see how you are travelling.

Not today, sweetie

Have a no-added-sugar day today.

Sugar does taste lovely but it robs your body of its nutrients, and encourages overeating, and so increases the chances of weight gain, heightens the risk of dental cavities and sharply increases the amount of insulin your body uses. Over time, this can heighten your risk of developing diabetes.

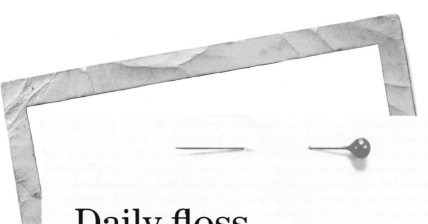

Daily floss

Floss your teeth today.
Give them a good clean-out.

We have all been told a million times we need to do it daily, but most of us don't. We know it will help to prevent decay and gum disease but it's so boring! We need to come to grips with this one. Flossing only takes 30 seconds after you brush your teeth and once you commit to it for a week or so, you realise just how much food and junk gets stuck between your teeth and gums even after you thoroughly brush.

Toilet training

Are you regular? Do you move your bowels every day?
Is it complete?
If you answered no to any of these questions, start some bowel training today.

It's just five steps:

1 Boost your high-fibre foods (whole grains, fruit and vegetables).
2 Increase your exercise—move it to move them.
3 Drink at least 2 litres (3½ pints) of water a day.
4 Relax! The bowels are where many of us hold on to emotional baggage and stress. Let it go.
5 Sit on the loo at the same time each day (morning is best) to remind your bowel of its job and allow your body to get into a regular rhythm. Give yourself time to go and time to finish.

An efficiently working bowel is a wonderful thing. Some people need to work harder than others to keep their bowel on its toes. For most of us, addressing the three cornerstones of good bowel health (exercise, water and fibre) is enough. Pay attention to your bowel health and you will be amazed at how it lifts your energy, spirits and wellbeing.

Bad habits

What is one habit you have that really annoys you?
Take a step towards breaking it today.

Sometimes committing to the first step is the biggest step of all.

Sore throat?

Here are your best natural weapons:

- An hourly gargle of 2 teaspoons salt in warm water, or 2 teaspoons lemon juice in warm water, or 2 tablespoons apple cider vinegar in a cup of warm water.
- A homemade tea of thyme or sage.

In *Culpepper's Complete Herbal* (1653), Culpepper said that thyme 'purgeth the body of phlegm'. It is also antiseptic and a local anaesthetic, making it excellent for soothing a sore or scratchy throat. Always spit out the gargle after using it and don't use salt if you have high blood pressure, or kidney or heart complaints.

Ordering your mind

Sit down and write out your weekly schedule today.
Write in all your activities
and those of your children and partner.
Break the day up into sections.
Find some time in there for you.
It may be a daily meditation session, some yoga,
reading time, an afternoon snooze or just sitting quietly
for five minutes.
Go on, pen it in so you make sure it happens.

Detoxing is about the mind, body and spirit. Clearing the clutter from your
mind is a fantastic way to detox, and writing a schedule transfers all of that
business from your head to paper. Writing a schedule can also show you
where you have gaps to fit in your chosen activities and relaxation time. If it
is written on a schedule, you are more likely to stick to it.

The phone boss

Be the boss of your phone.
Put the answering machine or message bank on today if you are really busy or having some time out.
Turn your phone off in the evening and don't turn it on again until 8 a.m.
Let the answering machine do some work. You can return the calls when you have the time and energy.

Technology is a great thing but it needs to be managed so that it works for us, not against us. Left unchecked, it steals our time and takes us away from what we intend to do. Keep it in its place so that you feel in control and able to manage your own time.

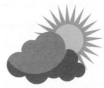

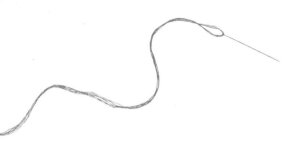

Eating discipline

Many of us rush our meals and eat on the run these days.
Bring yourself into the present when you are eating today.
It only takes an extra minute or two.
When you have a meal in front of you, smell it and look at it
before you eat it.
Take small mouthfuls and chew them well.
Really taste the food in your mouth. Feel the texture. Enjoy it.
Take time between mouthfuls to savour the meal.
Sit for a few minutes after the meal to rest and allow digestion
to begin.

On a physical level, good eating discipline enhances your digestion. On a
mental level, it satiates the appetite and feeds the brain. On a spiritual level,
it gives pleasure as you take the time to enjoy all aspects of your food, from
smell and taste to texture.

Sleepy byes

There is nothing better for our wellbeing
than a sound night's sleep.
If you are having trouble getting a good sleep,
try this drink tonight.
Warm a cup of milk on the stove.
Add 1 teaspoon honey and ½ teaspoon ground nutmeg.

This old-fashioned bedtime drink has some scientific support. Milk is rich in the amino acid tryptophan. Tryptophan converts to serotonin which has a lovely calming effect on the body. Nutmeg has the beautiful botanical name *Myristica frangrans*. It was a highly prized spice during medieval times and has a long history in the spices market. In small doses, it can be a calming sedative.

Quick warm snack

Try a new snack today.
Have miso soup for morning or afternoon tea.
It's an instant, nutritious snack and tastes delicious.
Miso soup is now widely available from Japanese
takeaways and as instant sachets from the supermarket,
or you can make it yourself from scratch using miso paste
and some fresh shallots. Simply mix a teaspoon or two of
the miso paste with a small amount of boiling water then
fill the cup with more boiling water and sprinkle on the
freshly chopped shallots.

Miso originated in China in 4BCE. It moved to Japan in 800CE and it
was thought that all who consumed it would enjoy health, happiness
and longevity—not a bad trio. It is made from fermented soy beans and
is a source of protein and other nutrients including zinc and B12. Miso
also contains an acidophilus-type substance which is great for digestive
disturbances.

Touch therapy

Ask your partner or one of your children to give you a shoulder rub.

It is not just the actual massage that is healing, but the touch. There is something very healing about the touch of someone who loves you. You feel it as a warmth, a glowing energy.

A pain in the butt

It's an embarrassing problem but if you suffer from piles or hemorrhoids, there are some natural ways to help ease and manage them. Try some of these simple remedies today and see what works for you.

- Boost the fibre in your diet.
- Drink at least two litres (3½ pints) of water a day.
- Run a warm, shallow bath, or buy a sitz bath, which allows you to sit comfortably, and add ½ cup of salt to it. Soak your bottom for 10–15 minutes to shrink the hemorrhoids and provide relief.
- Use damp toilet paper or flushable wipes when wiping yourself.
- Use a small amount of Hamamelis (witch hazel) cream on the area to help shrink them.

Hemorrhoids are a surprisingly common, painful problem for many women but one that is rarely discussed. It can be a result of poor diet, pregnancy or hereditary factors. Always consult your doctor if there is any bleeding or consistent pain and don't use the salt bath if you have any heart or kidney issues.

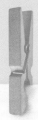

Herbal hydration

Find a new herbal tea you like today.
You may have never tried one or you may have a couple of favourites. Either way, find a new one to add to your repertoire.
Each cup of herbal tea you have adds to your total water intake for the day.
Chamomile is soothing and relaxing and lovely for the nerves.
Rosemary helps the memory and circulation.
Peppermint helps with wind and digestion.
Ginger is also good for digestion and circulation.

Unlike caffeinated tea, herbal tea is naturally caffeine-free and hydrates the body. Many of the blends have their own medicinal properties.

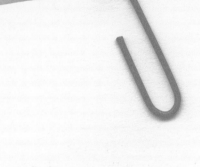

Love note

Write your partner a note telling them
five things you love about them.
Leave it somewhere you know they'll find it.

Simple, but we often forget the simple things and they are
always the best.

Out of touch

Can you touch your toes?
Give it a try right now.
Can you get past halfway?
Keep gently practising every day until you get there.
It will stretch everything out and keep everything moving.

The body is an amazing piece of engineering and design. Even if we have not done something for a long time, we can gently stretch and retrain muscles to do them once again. Get back in touch with your body and touch those toes.

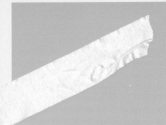

Cold blaster

Give this delicious smoothie a whirl today.
It will only take a few minutes to prepare.
Put these ingredients into your blender:
3 strawberries, 4 seeded and drained tinned guava cheeks,
½ cup frozen berries and ½ cup orange or cranberry juice.
Whiz until smooth.

This smoothie is packed with vitamin C, a cornerstone of any well-functioning immune system. Have this periodically throughout autumn and winter or at the very beginning of a cold to give your immunity a sharp boost. Make a double quantity if you have a child or partner who is a fussy eater. Most children love this delicious, sweet smoothie, so it is an excellent way to give their immune system a sneaky boost.

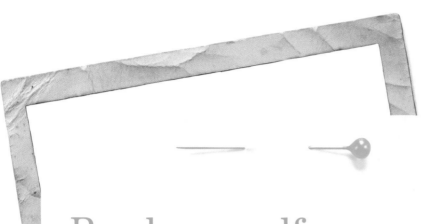

Read yourself

Make yourself a warm drink and sit down for five minutes and read the paper.

Sometimes it only takes five minutes to recentre ourselves and feel in control again. We are all busy, but you can always find five minutes. Learn to recognise your signals telling you that you need some time out to recentre, and take the few minutes you need. It may be a warm drink and the paper, five minutes alone in your room or even a short stint hiding in the work stationery cupboard. Whatever it takes, give yourself the time before it all comes crashing down.

Perfect posture

Next time you see a baby sitting on the floor, look at their beautiful natural poise—back straight, head aligned, shoulders down.

As you go about your day today, think about your own posture. When you sit at the computer, is everything relaxed and aligned? When you get the groceries out of the car, do you use your legs and not your back?

Think of your spine (back plus neck) and shoulders as a crucifix-shaped unit that is at the core of your posture. When they are aligned your muscles are relaxed, your spine is lengthened, your shoulders are broadened and you are in a relaxed and balanced state of rest.

Return to this balanced state of rest after every movement today and notice the profound effect it has on your stress and relaxation levels by the end of the day.

The Alexander technique focuses on achieving 'primary control' through retraining our posture or body alignment. It was developed by Matthias Alexander and was found to have therapeutic effects on movement, posture, respiration and tension patterns.

Sinus relief

If you have sore sinuses from the changeable autumn weather, press your thumbs on your face on either side of your nostrils and your index fingers between your eyebrows. Hold for a few seconds.
Repeat as necessary.

In traditional Chinese medicine, acupressure uses pressure on acupuncture points to help alleviate symptoms. Different symptoms are relieved by pressure on specific parts of the body.

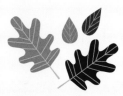

Dreaming

**Remember a dream you had as a child.
Can you make it come true?**

Life never turns out how we thought it would.
Sometimes we lose our way, forget ourselves
and discard our dreams. As a child, many of us
had great hopes and dreams. Take a minute
to remember yours. Do you still want it? Has it
changed? Can you make one of your dreams
come true? Life is short, it's worth thinking about.

Warm food energetics

Make warming foods the staple of your diet in these cooler months.
The best warming foods are:

- Vegetables—pumpkin, sweet potato or yam, leek, shallot, onion, squash, watercress
- Fruit—blackberry, peach, hawthorn, lychee, blackcurrant, cherry, quince
- Seeds and nuts—pine nut, pumpkin or pepita, sunflower, chestnut, walnut
- Herbs and spices—bay leaf, caraway seed, cardamom, chives, cinnamon, cloves, coriander, cumin, fennel seed, fenugreek, garlic, ginger, lemongrass, mustard, nutmeg, pepper, star anise

Food has a thermal or energetic nature. Some foods are naturally warming and so are great to include in our diet in autumn and winter. Warming foods move energy outwards and upwards from the centre of the body to the extremities. They warm us from the inside and help to galvanise us against infection.

Peace and quiet

Lie on a rug or mat as soon as you finish reading
this page.
Close your eyes.
Breathe in and out slowly.
Feel the breath reach the tips of your toes and fingers.
Imagine your breath is like a white light moving
through your body.
Slowly tense and relax every part of your body.
Start from the top of your head
and work to the soles of your feet.
Enjoy the peaceful state for five minutes.

Finding five minutes to relax and centre yourself can affect every aspect
of your life, from your health and relationships to your ability to think and
cope. It is a lovely habit to get into. If you talk to your children about it,
they may like to get into the habit too, or they may just respect your time
and leave you to it.

On the wagon

Drink no alcohol for the next three days.

Taken in moderation, some alcohol, such as red wine, has health benefits, but moderation is the key. Alcohol is packed with calories, has no nutrients, puts a strain on our liver and stimulates the biochemical pathways which can cause us to overeat. Try to give your body at least three consecutive alcohol-free days a week to rest your liver, reduce your calories and allow your body to regain its own natural rhythm.

House workout

Kill two birds with one stone today.
You don't have time to go to the gym
and you need to clean the house.
Do a house workout.
Put some dance music on and get to work.
Pick up the pace and dance while you are working up
a sweat.
Vaccuum with slightly bent knees to keep your thigh
muscles tight, dust using your whole shoulder, mop using
your torso as well as your arms, tighten your abdominals
as you polish and shine, and keep a smile on your face.

Regular exercise is difficult in our chaotic lives and so combining a
mundane necessity, such as cleaning the house, with exercise ticks
two boxes. Putting on some music and changing your mindset can
also make a very boring chore much more enjoyable.

Rubbing you the right way

Ever wondered about all of the different massages available these days?

Thai, kahuna, hot stone, remedial, Swedish, shiatsu—the delectable list goes on and on.

Do some research on them today and find a new and exciting one that you think suits you best.

If you like to be entertained while being massaged, choose kahuna. If you like it light and gentle, choose Swedish, or if you like a firm and therapeutic touch, perhaps remedial is the right one.

Be adventurous and book a new style for yourself this week or save up if you need to and book one as a reward.

Different styles of massage suit different people, depending on your symptoms and personality. Massage is not just an indulgence, it has a strong therapeutic effect and can ease aching muscles and, for some, reduce pain, stress and discomfort. If you are very interested in massage, many colleges and schools offer short courses. Your partner would be thrilled with your new skill.

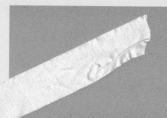

Wheat-free for a day

Make today a wheat-free day.
This means no bread, pasta, cakes, biscuits, anything that
contains wheat.
Replace it with rice, spelt, barley, oats, rye or any other grain.
You could try porridge for breakfast, stir-fry with steamed rice
for lunch and a salad for dinner.

Many of us eat wheat at every meal. Due to this overload, many develop
an intolerance, so after eating wheat we feel bloated, windy or just
uncomfortable. Giving your body a rest from it can help to reduce the
symptoms. You may be surprised how good you feel when not eating
wheat. It is a hard habit to break as most of our convenience foods are
made with our favourite grain. It is worth persisting as once the habit is
broken, eating wheat-free foods becomes second nature.

Head banging

The autumn winds give many of us headaches.
Before you reach for the paracetamol, try this.
Press a finger between your eyebrows and hold.
If no relief, place a finger either side of the webbing
between your thumb and index finger.
Apply pressure and hold.

These two points are the acupressure points for general headaches and
when pressure is applied they can help to reduce the severity of the pain
without the use of drugs. It's free and it's easy, so it's worth a try.

Rebuilding your strength

At this cooling time of year, you may be recovering from an illness, so take some time today to make some barley water and sip it throughout the day.

Barley water is made by adding 1 cup unrefined barley to 2 litres (3½ pints) water. Boil in a large pot for about three hours and then strain. Discard the barley and sip the barley water or broth throughout the day. If you still have a sore throat or digestive upset, add some powdered slippery elm as it will soothe these areas.

Drinking barley water is an ancient practice. It is highly nutritive and is used to rebuild or fortify a person's strength after illness. It is also very useful if you suffer from cystitis. It can be flavoured with lemon or honey. For extra flavour you could add some lemon rind to the water while it is boiling.

Saying sorry

Say sorry to someone you have wronged in the past.

Sorry is such a powerful word. Saying sorry takes courage, strength and humility, and you are the greatest winner as you no longer have to harbour the memory or the feelings of what you did. You are free and so are they.

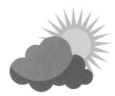

Full steam ahead

Buy a vegetable steamer today
or write it on your shopping list to buy soon.
Use it every time you cook vegetables.

If you boil vegetables you lose 50 per cent of their vitamins and minerals. If you steam, you lose a measly 15 per cent. Steaming is an amazing way to give your diet a multivitamin and mineral lift. If you have children, it is even more important to steam as children are often fussy about eating vegetables and so those they do eat need to be as nutritious as possible.

A detox bath

Tonight is just the night for a detox bath.
Let's flush out those lingering toxins that are holding
you back from being your best.
Run a warm bath and add 2 cups apple cider vinegar
and 2 drops rosemary essential oil.
Soak until the water cools, then pat yourself dry.

Apple cider vinegar is deeply detoxifying and will also soothe itchy or irritated
skin. Rosemary essential oil detoxes the mind by clearing out the clutter.
It works on the body by stimulating and strengthening the liver and respiratory
system, and encouraging the flow of bile.
Don't use the rosemary essential oil if you are pregnant or suffer from epilepsy.

Honey, honey

Gently warm 2 tablespoons honey.
Smear the warm honey onto your face.
Leave for 2–3 minutes or until the honey begins to 'pull'.
Rinse off and pat your skin dry.

Honey is a natural, gentle, instant cleanser
that leaves the skin clean and soft.

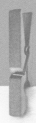

Get a hobby

What are you interested in?
Photography, painting, sewing, gardening, makeup, cooking?
Do some research into it and join a group, find a specialist
shop, or find friends with a similar interest and meet up.
Take it up as a hobby.

Hobby is such an old-fashioned, daggy word, but it is a wonderful way
to enrich your life and develop your own sense of self. For single people,
it is also an excellent way to meet new people and broaden your world.
It gives you something just for yourself beyond your family, duties and
obligations, and so connects you to your true self.

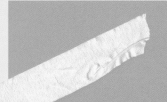

Odourless underarms

The sun of summer has faded and so we are less sweaty and hot.
Unless you suffer from strong body odour, you don't need strong chemical deodorants through the cooler months.
For autumn and winter, switch to a natural aluminium-free alternative.
Check the labels on the deodorants in the health food shop or supermarket, or try a crystal. It sounds strange but they can work a treat on some people and are all natural and totally chemical free.

Most commercial deodorants contain the metal aluminium amongst numerous other chemicals. Switching to an all-natural deodorant, if only during the colder months, is just another way of reducing the chemical load you place on your body.

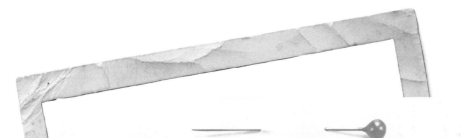

In the white of the eye

Take a close look at your sclera, the white of your eye, today.
Gently pull up the lid of one eye so you can clearly see the white
of the eye above the iris.
Check for the presence of red lines at the top of the eyes.
This is where stress and nervous strain is indicated on the sclera.
The more numerous the red lines, the more intense the stress and
strain you are under.
If there are many lines present, work on a stress management
plan today, and find some simple things you can do regularly to
actively manage your stress.

Sclerology, an ancient diagnostic art, is the study of the red lines in the white
of the eyes and how they relate to stress patterns in a person's health. If this
interests you, go online and download a sclerology map and 'read' your eyes,
or search for a sclerology practitioner near you.

Tea time

Try a new tea today.
It is called 'rooibos' and is widely available from health food stores and supermarkets.
Replace every second cup of coffee or tea for the day with rooibos.
Make it just like normal tea, adding milk and honey as you desire.

Rooibos, meaning 'red bush' in Africaans, is a traditional South African tea which tastes very similar to our usual black tea but has many wonderful health benefits. It is naturally caffeine-free, anti-inflammatory, antiviral and contains more polyphenols than green tea, making it a fantastic antioxidant. It is also excellent for digestion, managing the appetite, sleep and calming shaky nerves. After a long, hard day two of the cold, wet teabags make a wonderful eye mask!

Help me

If you need some help today, ask for it.

How often do you struggle with organising things, running around, carrying too much, lifting something too heavy, worrying about everyone and never asking for help? Today is the day to ask for it. It's not hard to do and is a good habit to get in to. You will get the help you need and the person helping you will feel good about themselves—a win-win situation.

Sweet enough

Check your food labels today.
Just how much sugar is in your yoghurt, soft drink or muesli bar?
Sugar can appear as sugar, sucrose, glucose, fructose, fructose syrup, maltose, corn syrup, honey, molasses, maple syrup, invert sugar, dextrose, golden syrup, lactose, malt or maltose. Fancy names but to your body they all mean sugar.
You'll be surprised how easy it is to cut your sugar without cutting your taste.
Slowly reducing it over time will allow your tastebuds to adjust and you will not miss the additional sweetness.

Sugar is hidden in many processed and supermarket-bought foods. The maximum you should have is about 2–3 teaspoons of sugar per serve. Make the switch to brands that are lower in sugar and save those extra calories sitting on your hips.

Tired brains

Make this massage oil today for those days when your mind aches and your mental batteries are flat. To a 100 millimetre (3½ fluid ounce) bottle of almond oil, add 10 drops lavender essential oil, 10 drops geranium essential oil, 4 drops peppermint essential oil and 15 drops chamomile oil.
Give it a gentle shake and store it in a cool, dark place ready to recharge your batteries when you need it.

It is good practice to add the contents of two vitamin E capsules to your massage oils. It will not only make them even better for your skin, it will also help to preserve them and protect them from going rancid.

Call your family

Call someone in your family today.
Make it someone you haven't spoken to in a while.
Have a chat with them and reconnect.

Time flies and we get caught up in the everyday,
letting some of our important connections slip.
Reconnecting with someone close to you can help
you feel loved and supported.

Someone else's shoes

Think about someone close to you.
It may be your partner, child, best friend, mum or sister.
Take a minute to walk in their shoes.
How do things look from their point of view?
Would you change anything if you were them?
Can you make any changes to improve your relationship
with them?

We always see things through our own eyes, often not understanding
where someone close to us is coming from. This gap can be damaging to a
relationship, so take the time to walk in their shoes and see how things look for
them. It may give you a much greater understanding.

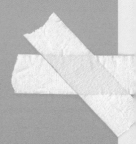

Brush your skin

Before showering today, give your skin a vigorous brush with a pure bristle dry skin brush. Starting with the soles of your feet, brush your entire body. Always brush upwards towards the heart. It will make you feel invigorated and alive.

Dry skin brushing is a fantastic naturopathic practice, because it stimulates your circulation and the lymphatic system, removes dead skin and encourages cell renewal, leaving your skin glowing with vitality. You can buy dry skin brushes from most health food stores and homeware shops.

You are what you eat

Use one of the cookbooks gathering dust on your shelf
and find a healthy new dish for dinner.
Add it to your family's dinner repertoire today, and drop
an unhealthy one.

As queen of the kitchen, you are a key contributor to your health
and wellbeing and that of your family. Changing your dinner choices
can have a marked effect on everyone's health, behaviour, energy
levels and sleep. Relentless as it may be, cooking is the highest art
and a cornerstone of a happy, healthy household. Are there some
simple choices you could make to give your family a boost?

Social networking

How are things in the friends department?
Do you have enough to support you, encourage you and have fun with?
Do you have too many to be able to foster close and connected friendships?

Taking stock of our social lives can help us to rebalance things and encourage us to invest time into areas where we need to. Friends play a huge role in how we feel about ourselves and how we cope with our everyday lives. If the balance is right, life can be a whole lot easier and enjoyable.

Your cycle

Start a menstrual calendar in your diary today.
Write down when you begin and end your period and
any notable symptoms before, during and after.

The regularity and pattern of your cycle tells much about how your body
is functioning. Once you have filled in the calendar for a few months,
check to see the length of your cycle, the regularity, the consistency of
symptoms. If there are any irregularities or persistent discomfort, make an
appointment to see your healthcare professional.

Recovery plan

If you are feeling under the weather today or recovering from an illness, write down three things you can do over the next week to allow your body to rest, recuperate and fight any lingering bugs.
List simple things like drink fresh ginger tea, rest, and accept help when it is offered.

Convalescence is an old-fashioned term still used by naturopaths because it's so important. Everyone needs time to recover from an illness, big or small. In our grandmothers' time, it was accepted as part of life. Now we 'soldier on', which isn't that smart, so take stock and give yourself time to get back on your feet.

Take the plunge

Is there something important that you really need in one of your relationships that you are not getting? Choose your time well and in a calm and considered way, ask for it today.

Sometimes we forget to just ask for things. The people in our lives are not mind readers and although something looks obvious to us, it may be nowhere on the radar for the other person. Do you need some praise from your mum? Would you like your partner to tell you they love you? Would you like your friend to decide where you are going out on the weekend for a change? Whatever it is that you need, consider it and gently ask the person for it. You may be surprised by how happy they are to give it to you.

Warming oil

Add 2 cloves of fresh garlic and a knob of fresh ginger to your olive oil. Leave the oil for a month and it will be ready for your winter cooking.

Garlic is antibiotic, antibacterial and antiseptic. It's a great tonic for the digestion, the heart and the respiratory system. Ginger is wonderful for aches and pains and very warming. These herbs will infuse the oil with their therapeutic properties, which will give all of your winter cooking extra warmth and health.

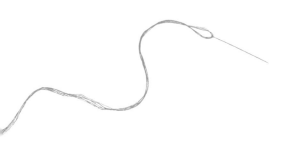

Revive your feet

Run a small bath or fill a bucket with warm water.
Add some lavender essential oil and some fresh or
dried mint leaves.
Soak your feet for ten minutes while you help with
homework, read to your child, make a list, think about
the day or, best of all, just relax.

There is something incredibly relaxing about soaking your feet in a
bucket of water, with or without essential oils. It gives you five minutes
for yourself, cares for your hard-working feet and gives you perspective
on your day, all for next to nothing.

Focus on your breath

Lay on a rug or mat, close your eyes and breathe in and out slowly. Slowly tense and then relax every part of your body from the top of your head to the tip of your toes. Free your worries and enjoy five minutes in this peaceful state.

Slowly tensing and relaxing each part of your body can help to make you more aware of where you are holding tension and stress. Sometimes we are more tense, stressed or exhausted than we realise. This exercise can give you a reality check of how you are travelling.

Tasty treat

Winter is around the corner, so let's give your immune system a treat today.

Make this easy snack so you can have a treat and give your immune system a boost at the same time.

Mix together ½ cup of each of the following ingredients: dried blackcurrants, roughly chopped dried apricots, roughly chopped dried peaches, almonds, sunflower seeds and pepitas.

Store in an airtight jar.

Important nutrients for the immune system are vitamins A, C and E and the mineral zinc. The yummy snack above is rich in all of these and is a wonderful way to give your immune system a 'shot in the arm'. It is also a highly nutritious snack for children. If there are any nut allergies in the family, omit the nuts.

Winter

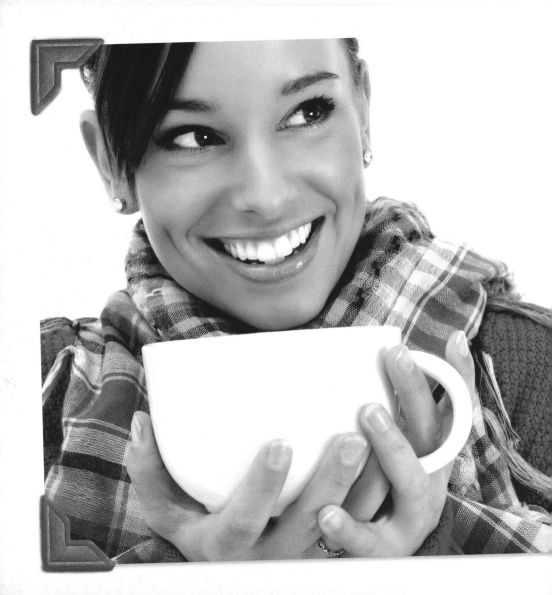

The cold, chilly season, with its beautiful bare trees and bracing air, offers us an intimacy the other seasons do not. We spend more time inside with family and friends —chatting at the dinner table, enjoying the crackle of an open fire, or tucked up and cosy in bed. The warmth of the home replaces the warmth of the sun.

Nature conserves her energy as many animals, trees and plants sleep through the long, cold months ready to be woken for the spring once again.

Winter diet

The chills of winter are once again upon us.
We need to take extra care to keep ourselves warm.
One way to do this is through our diet.
Time to change to your warming winter diet.
Stop eating raw or cold foods and pull out the slow cooker.
Move to a warm, well-cooked diet filled with soups, stews,
casseroles and tagines.

Winter brings with it the cold, wind and rain. It can be a beautiful time
of year but we need to take extra care of ourselves to ensure we stay
strong and well. Pack your meals with the best of the warming winter
vegetables, the root vegetables. This includes swedes, turnips, potatoes,
sweet potato and pumpkin.

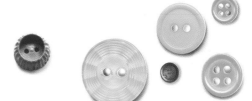

Just for you

When was the last time you did something just for you?
After the children are tucked up in bed tonight, run
a bubble bath, add a few drops of your favourite
essential oils and light some candles.

The simple act of soaking in the bath can wash the stresses of the day
away, reconnect you with your spirit, and give you time and space away
from the demanding job of being you.

Ear rub

Sit comfortably with your back straight.
Use your thumbs and index fingers to rub and
gently pull your ears from the top to bottom.
Repeat for a minute on each ear.

Just like the feet, the ears contain reflexology areas
and points corresponding to major body parts and
areas. Giving them an all-over rub can help to improve
circulation and the flow of chi (life energy) throughout
the body. Rubbing your ears may look strange but it is
highly therapeutic and relaxing.

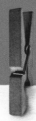

Winter solstice

Look up on the internet or your calendar
the date of this year's winter solstice.
Mark it in your diary.
Plan a small ceremony to celebrate the solstice and be
thankful for the gift of another winter with the beauty of
spring just around the corner.

'O, wind if Winter comes, can Spring be far behind?' wrote the famous
poet Shelley. Indeed the winter solstice, the shortest day of the year,
can be dark and grey but winter has a character and intimacy all its own.
Enjoy it on the winter solstice, knowing the flowers of spring are soon to
raise their faces to the sun.

Beat the cold

Have you woken feeling a little under the weather this morning?
Congestion can make us feel foggy and unable to think clearly.
Put a few drops of eucalyptus or Breathe Easy oil on a handkerchief or burn it in an oil burner.
It will help to clear your sinuses and so sharpen your thinking, making you more productive and able to enjoy the day.

Eucalyptus oil is a powerful antiseptic and cleanser. It is wonderful for colds, coughs and other winter ills, and it crystallises the mind. Put a few drops in a spritz bottle with some water and spray liberally around a room to clear negative energy or to cleanse the room after someone has recovered from illness.

Think positive

This is a day to think positively.
Negative thought patterns are often the seed
of unhappiness.
Banish them today by talking over them with a mantra.

A mantra is a positive phrase, word or sound you say over and over
in your mind. It may be 'I deserve good things in my life' or 'I am a
capable, wonderful woman'. Over time, the mantra begins to work its
magic and you believe what you are repeating, leaving no space for
the negative.

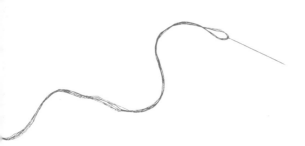

Chesty cough

If you have a chesty winter cough, make up this simple chest rub today.
Stir together 2 drops each of tea tree oil, lavender essential oil and rosemary essential oil with 1 teaspoon vegetable or jojoba oil.
Massage onto the chest area.

This combination of oils is soothing, warming, antiseptic and helps to break down mucus. Massaging onto the chest area also creates warmth in the area and allows the odour of the oils to be smelt throughout the day, thereby increasing their therapeutic effect.

No more windy days

Feeling bloated, windy or uncomfortable after you eat?
Give your digestive system a treat today with a digestive
herbal tea.
Try some mint, chamomile, fennel or lemon balm on their
own or in a blend.
These herbs have wonderful properties that can help ease
indigestion, wind and nausea and, if drunk regularly, will
help promote good digestion.

Good digestion is the cornerstone of good health, and some people
have to work harder at it than others. Teas made with good-quality
herbs can be an excellent way to promote good digestion and ease
feelings of discomfort. Be adventurous and try something new or buy
a digestive blend.

Winter warmer

Make a big pot of vegetable soup for dinner tonight.
Your challenge is to pack in as many different
vegetables as you can.
Can you get the count up to ten?

A big pot of vegetable soup is like a multivitamin meal that helps to
fortify us in winter. It is rich in all of the vitamins and minerals our bodies
need to fight the winter bugs. Make a large pot and freeze what you
don't eat in meal-sized portions.

Do a friend audit

Think about which of your friends are zappers (give you energy and make you feel good) and which of your friends are sappers (take your energy and make you feel bad). Make a decision to spend more time with the zappers.

The people in your close circle have a great influence on the way you think and feel about your life, your family and yourself. We don't always take the time to think about how healthy our friendships are. Spending more time with the friends who make you feel happy, comfortable and alive can have a wonderful effect on your wellbeing.

Banish aches and pains

You know those days when you seem to be 'in the wars'.
You bump into this, knock into that, everything seems to be
in the way.
Get out some arnica cream or ointment.
It will bring out your bruises, help you heal faster, and will
ease aches, pains, bruises and sprains. It is also great for
those aching varicose veins.

Arnica Montana is a herb in the same family as soothing chamomile or the
healing calendula. It has many therapeutic properties, helping to promote
healing and reduce pain. Use it topically and not for prolonged periods, just for
those times when you are feeling knocked about or your aching legs won't let
you sleep.

Rest

Lie on the bed for half an hour today
and read a book or watch TV.
It will make no difference to the house if you
take 30 minutes for yourself.
The washing is not going anywhere and the
dishes will wait.

As a woman, you give a great deal to other people with little
thought for your own needs. Your list of jobs never seems to
end. Taking some time for yourself has two benefits; it gives
your body a rest from your very physically demanding job,
and reminds you that you deserve to have your needs met
just like everyone else in the family.

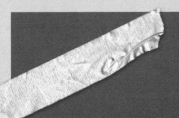

Sinus blast

Winter and congestion go hand in hand.
If you are feeling a little congested today, before you reach
for the pills, reach inside the fridge instead.
See if you can find a jar of horseradish.
It is a great way to clear your sinuses naturally.
Take a small amount to check that you can tolerate it and
then work up to a ¼ teaspoon.
Use it each time your sinuses begin to block.

Armoracia rusticana or horseradish has been cultivated since antiquity. It is in
the same family as mustard, wasabi, broccoli and cabbage, and is an excellent
decongestant and circulatory stimulant. It is a fantastic natural way to quickly
clear congestion. It is super hot, so proceed with caution and miss it altogether
if you are pregnant.

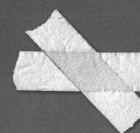

A winter flame

Get your oil burner out today and drop in a winter blend.

Add 3 drops each of cedarwood, rosemary and clove essential oils.

Carefully top it up with some boiling water and light the candle to enjoy the lovely smells of winter.

Blend as you go or make a small bottle of the blend to use throughout the winter. If you have only one or two of the oils, it will work just as well.

Give to receive

'Winter is on my head, but eternal spring is in my heart.' Victor Hugo
Commit to supporting one charity
that you believe in.
It may be a time donation or a money donation.
Every bit helps.

It is not the amount but the intent that will rekindle your spirit.

Warm from the inside

Start with a warm breakfast today
to steel you against a cold winter's day.
Combine some winter fruit with a small amount of
apple juice and a stick or pinch of cinnamon.
Gently simmer until warm and just softened.
Serve with room-temperature natural yoghurt.

Warm food for breakfast in winter can help to fuel the digestive fire for
the rest of the day. It warms you from the inside and keeps the winter
cold at bay.

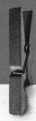

Get your winter fires burning

Buy some Mu tea today or make a pot of herbal tea with cinnamon, licorice or ginseng.
Keep it warm and sip it through the day.

These herbs all help to warm the body and get your digestive fires burning in preparation for the cold of winter. The Mu tea blend is good for the blood, invigorating your chi or life energy. It's great when you are feeling lethargic. You can re-use the tea bags a number of times and even make a half tea, half apple juice drink from them. This will be a favourite with your kids.

Open yourself

Accept help when it is offered today.

You may be used to saying 'No, I'm ok' before even thinking about it. If help is offered today, accept it. There is nothing wrong with lightening your load and letting someone make your life a little easier. It can be as rewarding for them as it is for you.

First line of winter defence

Can you feel your throat getting scratchy, or your nose blocking up?
Is a cough creeping up on you?
Here is your first line of winter defence: vitamin C, garlic tablets and echinacea tincture or tablets.
This little army will stop most colds before they progress, if you act as soon as you feel them begin.

Vitamin C is a fantastic way to boost your immune system naturally. Garlic contains an active component called allicin which is antiseptic, antibacterial, antifungal and helps to break down mucus, making it easier to expel from the body. Echinacea is antiseptic and antiviral. It gives the immune system a wonderful boost. The combination of the three is formidable to infections. Dose regularly as per the recommendation on the pack.

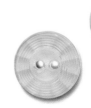

A clean, healthy house for next to nothing

Take a minute and have a look at your cleaning products.
For not much money, many of them can be replaced by these four
cheap, effective and natural alternatives:

- Salt—antiseptic, disinfectant and a great scouring agent
- White vinegar—cuts through grease and soap residue,
  antimould, mild disinfectant, deodorant, bleach,
  all-purpose cleaner
- Lemons—mild bleach, deodorant, cleaning agent
- Bicarbonate of soda—stain remover, water softener, polish,
  scourer, removes unpleasant odours.

Every day we are exposed to thousands of chemicals in our own home. Reducing
the potentially harmful chemicals in your cleaning cupboard by downsizing and
going natural is an excellent way to reduce your everyday chemical exposure,
cut your cleaning bill and also contribute to a sustainable environment.

Friendly quiz

How well do you know your friends?
How well do they know you?
Take some time today to find out a few things about
your friends that you never knew.

Intimate connections to our family and friends help us to feel loved,
valued, supported and nurtured. They are a privilege, not a right and
so need some time, love and effort to be developed and deepened.
Regularly checking in with the health of your close relationships is a
great way to consider your own emotional health.

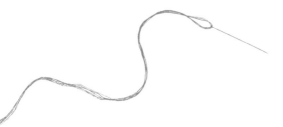

A teaspoon a day

In a ceramic bowl, mix together 1 teaspoon each of ground clove, nutmeg and cinnamon, 2 teaspoons each of dried peppermint, sage and rosemary, 2 teaspoons crushed garlic, and 1 litre (1¾ pints) apple cider vinegar.
Place mixture in a glass jar and seal tightly.
Leave in strong sunlight for fifteen days to allow it to steep, then strain it, bottle it and store it in a cool, dark place.
You now have the once highly prized 'Four Thieves Vinegar'.
Take 1 teaspoon a day through winter to ward off ills, add it to your bathwater to keep you protected and safe, or use it as a general disinfectant throughout the house.

Four Thieves Vinegar has a fascinating history and many variations.
It is said that in the 1630s, when the Black Plague was raging through France, four thieves invented a herbal disinfectant that would protect them so they could rob without fear of infection.
It worked very well and when they were finally arrested in Toulouse, the judge offered them a deal and the four thieves traded their recipe in return for a merciful death.

Go for a dip

You know those dangerous times of day when you are absolutely ravenous and eat too much of the wrong things before you know what's happened? Those famished frenzies can undo all of your good work. Take a few minutes today to work out some simple, delicious and healthy snacks you can have on hand for those ravenous times. A great one is a bowl of healthy dip like homemade hommus kept in the fridge with some cut-up vegetable sticks.

To make hommus, put these ingredients into a blender. 1 tin (400 grams/14 ounces) rinsed and drained chick peas, 3 tablespoons tahini, 2 cloves garlic, 2 tablespoons extra virgin olive oil, and the juice of 2 or 3 lemons (to taste). Whiz until smooth and keep it in the fridge in an airtight container.

Having healthy, instant and delicious snacks on hand can add some great foods to your diet and, importantly, take the danger out of those hunger pangs.

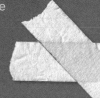

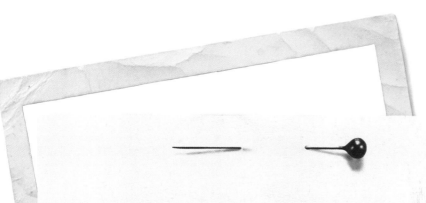

A kidney warmer

Get warm from the inside tonight.
Heat 2 cups of salt and carefully pour it into an old pillowcase.
Wrap it tightly.
Place the warm salt bag against your kidneys (lower back) and rest against the back of a chair.
Remove the bag if it becomes too hot or uncomfortable.
Feel the warmth build within you.

Traditionally, warmth enters and exits the body through the kidney area in our lower back. Applying this gentle heat to the area will help to invite warmth into your body.

Clean underwear

Clean out your underwear drawer today. Throw out anything your mother (or grandmother) would consider wearing, anything with holes in it and anything that suffers from sagginess.

Foxy undies don't have to cost the earth and they make you feel great! Wearing saggy old knickers, something we have all been guilty of at one time or another, looks awful and makes you feel pretty shabby too. Of course, we all remember what Mum said about wearing good underwear in case of an accident. I don't know if she was expecting us to meet a dreamy ambo…

Cold clearer

Add something new to your winter first aid kit today.
Buy some Kali Mur Glandular tonic.
It's great for helping to clear congestion,
coughs and sore throats.
Start dosing, as per the instructions on the label,
at the first sign of symptoms.

Kali Mur is a tissue salt. Tissue salts are homeopathic remedies and their therapeutic properties have been used since the nineteenth century. Homeopathy means 'like cures like' so a disease or symptom set is treated with medicines made from the materials that cause similar signs and symptoms in a healthy person. From the beginning of the reign of Queen Victoria until the present day, the British royal family use the services of a homeopathic physician to support their health and wellbeing.

Hand treatment

Today you're making a natural hand cream to get rid of that winter crocodile skin.

Place an egg yolk and 1 teaspoon fresh lemon juice into the blender and whiz.

Slowly add ⅓ cup of vegetable or almond oil, ¼ cup sunflower oil and 5 drops of your favourite essential oil.

Once it is thick and creamy, place it into a glass jar and keep it in the fridge.

Rub it on your hands whenever you think of it.

Winter is very drying for your skin and dry hands can make you feel old and wrinkly! This combination of oils, egg and lemon is soothing to dry skin and helps to heal and protect it from the harshness of winter.

Kidney tune-up

Winter is the season of the kidney.
In traditional Chinese medicine, the emotion attached to our kidneys is fear and anxiety and the health of the kidneys determines our longevity.
With good kidney energy you will be grounded and dependable.
If your kidney energy is out of balance, you will run from problems rather than resolve them, and feel that life is just too hard. You always feel tired.
In children, chronic bedwetting can be the kidney subconsciously expressing fear.

If the emotions attached to your kidneys are out of balance, boost your kidney-friendly foods including walnuts, parsley, shallots, leeks, pepper, seeds, black beans, kidney beans and blueberries. Take a break from the stimulation of media and technology and schedule a quiet day of contemplation to recentre yourself and allow your kidney energy to begin to flow freely again.

Dear diary

Have you ever thought about keeping a diary? They don't have to start at the beginning of the year. Why not start one now while you are rugged up inside for winter.

Diaries or journals can be an excellent way to express your creative self, sort out your feelings, allow time for introspection, and give you a different perspective on your life and direction.

Liver tonic

Get your juicer out today and take five minutes to whip up this liver tonic.
Juice 3 carrots, ¼ beetroot and 2 stalks of celery. Drink immediately.

Carrots and beetroot are both rich in beta-carotene (a form of vitamin A) and carotenoids making them excellent anti-cancer foods and liver lovers. Celery is a good source of folate, potassium, manganese and vitamin C, and helps cleanse the liver by supporting the kidneys. This drink is also a great immune booster.

Winter wonder food

Your superfood for today is shiitake mushrooms.
Use them instead of normal mushrooms in your
dinner tonight.

Shiitake mushrooms have long been used in traditional Chinese medicine
for increasing resistance to infection and supporting the immune system.
They are a medicinal wonderfood and are now widely available in fruit and
vegetable shops. Adding them to your dishes will really boost nutrition and
your immune system to keep you well throughout the winter.

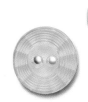

Learn something new today

Go online today and look up something that you know nothing about.
Something like geography, politics, maths, birthstones, astrology or astronomy.
Learn some key facts about it.
Make that brain work out a little.

Most of us use school as a marker of our intelligence. If we didn't get good grades, we resign ourselves to not being very smart. This pigeonholing can play quite a role in our lives, limiting us and eroding our confidence. Park these labels. Stretch your brain and challenge it with new things. The online world gives us instant access to a world of information, use it. Become an expert in something you love. Feed your brain and it will reward you with confidence in your own ability.

Eat chocolate!

Eat some chocolate today, but not all day.
Make it the best quality chocolate.
That means dark chocolate made by a
reputable company.

Dark chocolate has a larger concentration of beneficial
nutrients and less sugar and fillers than milk chocolate.
Research shows that the active component of dark
chocolate, theobromine, has positive effects on
your cardiovascular and respiratory systems. Eat it in
moderation, though. A couple of squares should nip a
craving in the bud.

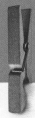

Triggering relaxation

Relax yourself in a moment today.
Use your middle fingers to feel beside each eyebrow for the slight depression in your skull (your temples).
Apply gentle, rotating pressure.
Now place the heel of your left hand on your right collarbone. Rest your thumb against your neck and allow your fingers to go over your shoulder and rest. The resting place of your middle finger is your second trigger point.
Apply firm pressure while tapping your middle finger.

These are two of your relaxation trigger points. Find them this morning and use them throughout the day for instant relaxation.

Pumpkin power

The superfood for today is pumpkin.
Roast it, steam it, puree it or bake it
but eat some today.
It is great in soups, stews, warm in salads or
mashed with other orange vegetables.

Pumpkin is high in vitamins C and E, potassium, magnesium
and beta-carotene. It is great for the eyes, skin, immune
system and blood.

Colour your world red

Wear some red today.
It may be a complete outfit, a coat or just a scarf.
As long as it is visible to the world.
It will change your outlook on the day.

In colour therapy, red is warm and stimulating.
It is daring and increases energy and passion.
It helps with circulation and energises our
senses. Working its magic on our first chakra,
it can also stimulate sexual energy.

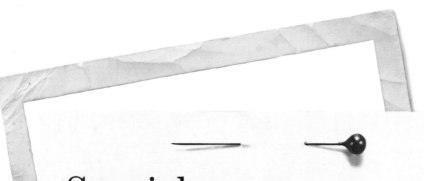

Special space

Find a place today where you feel peaceful and calm.
A place where you can relax and reconnect with yourself.
It can be a place at home, at work, at the park or even a
place in your mind.
Go to or think of this space when you are feeling agitated,
annoyed or stressed.

It can be hard to recentre ourselves in the middle of our chaotic lives. Having
a special space or place where you know you can retreat can help you to
immediately connect with those feelings of peace and harmony that melt away
stress and tension.

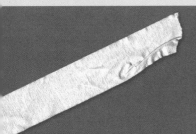

Cold hands, warm heart

A lovely saying, but cold hands
can be painful in the winter months.
Make some fresh ginger tea this morning by chopping
a knob of fresh ginger and gently simmering it in some
boiling water for two minutes.
Place it in a thermos and sip it throughout the day.
It will warm you through.
Try to have it half an hour before meals to get the
digestive fires burning before you eat.

Ginger or *Zingiber officinalis* is used by naturopaths and herbalists to
promote circulation. One of the advantages of moving your warm blood
around faster and more efficiently is that you stay warmer, especially in
your hands and feet.

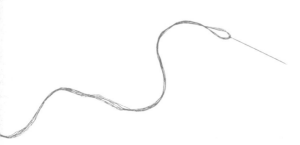

Funny medicine

When was the last time you laughed so hard you cried?
Remember how good you felt afterwards.
Think about what makes you laugh.
Is it a book, a person, a show, a song, a movie, YouTube
videos, a joke?
Think of what makes you laugh and make an effort today
to connect to it and get giggly.

Laughter therapy actually uses laughter as a therapeutic tool. We are
born knowing how to laugh but we learn to be serious. For many of us,
the older we grow, the more serious we become. Laughter comes from
deep within us and works its magic helping us to feel better, change our
perspective and see things more clearly.

Clove tea

Drop a couple of cloves into your tea this morning.
If you like it, stick with it through the cold months until
the sunshine of spring is once again upon us.

The deep distinctive smell of clove raises the spirits. In ancient
Chinese medical scripts, the clove is one of the earliest medicinal
herbs mentioned. In the fifteenth century, it was one of the most
precious and expensive spices in the world. In the herbal classic,
A Modern Herbal (1931), Mrs Maud Grieves tells us that cloves are
used for nausea, flatulence and indigestion. The wonderful clove
is also a powerful antiseptic, germicide, disinfectant, antibacterial,
antifungal and antiviral and so is a beneficial addition to your winter
tea. For a toothache, put a few drops of clove oil onto a clean piece
of cloth and position it between the tooth and the gums.

Change just one thing

You may have many stressors in your life
and feel overwhelmed.
Today, change just one thing.
It may be preparing dinner in the morning to avoid the
evening rush, having lunch with someone who makes you
laugh, organising to have your bills paid automatically
online, or writing up a weekly schedule.
Just one thing can make a big difference.

Change can be difficult but breaking problems down into smaller
pieces and then dealing with them makes it more manageable.
Sometimes, just relieving stress in one area can have a great knock-
on effect in other areas, and once you have made one change
successfully, you may be willing to introduce another.

Seated tilts

If you are sitting for long periods today, perhaps at a desk or driving, give your lower back a relaxing workout with some pelvic tilts. Every 20–30 minutes, tilt your pelvis back and forward five times.

The lower back can become stiff and sore when held in the same position for long periods of time, such as when you are working at a desk or driving a long distance. Moving your pelvis helps to mobilise and relieve pressure in this problem spot.

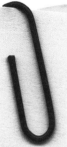

Exciting plans

It's fun to get excited about something, to look forward to it.

Plan something for this Saturday night.

It doesn't have to be big budget, just a little different to your usual routine.

A family pizza night, a quiet movie with popcorn for two, a date with your partner, a friend for dinner.

Life can become mundane with days all feeling the same. You get bored and start to tune out. Planning something special can spark your imagination, lift your spirits and engage you with those around you.

Body language

Just like your diet and lifestyle, your thoughts and emotions play a major role in your health.

Take a moment to consider if your thoughts and emotions are playing a positive or a negative role.

What could you do to express them more freely?

Do you need to have a chat to a professional to help unravel and understand them?

Make a pledge to yourself to have more positive thoughts than negative for the day and notice the effect it has on you as your day progresses.

Research has shown the hormones and neurotransmitters (the body's messengers) effect the immune system and that the immune system also effects the brain. So every thought, feeling or mood we experience triggers the release of chemical messengers, which communicate our moods and feelings to our body. Listen to what your thoughts and feelings are but also listen to the language of your body.

The vagueness of the vagus

If you are watching your weight, have smaller meals today. Wait at least ten minutes until you have 'seconds'.

Along with other helpers, there is a nerve in the body called the vagus nerve that tells our brains when we are full. It has many vital functions including regulating our heartbeat and keeping us breathing. The 'being full' message is a long way down on the list, so even when we have had enough food, it takes a while for the message to get to the brain and make us feel full. So waiting ten minutes after you eat gives your vagus the chance to get its messages delivered and helps you to resist that second serve of lasagne.

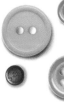

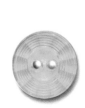

Make the call

'One kind word can warm three winter months.'
Japanese proverb
Call someone who makes you feel great today.

There are some people who make us feel great.
They just give you that little spring in your step and bring a smile
to your face. They bring out the best in you.
It only takes five minutes to give them a quick call and it can make
your day and theirs.

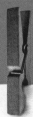

Bid the chill goodbye

It is an old-fashioned term, but sometimes you feel like you have a chill.
If you are feeling like that today, try this ginger warmer.
Grate or finely chop 1½ cups fresh ginger.
Place it in a rectangular shape in the middle of a clean tea towel or
pillowcase and wrap it up, making a rectangle. It should look like one of
those wheat bags.
Place it in a saucepan and pour over just enough boiling water to cover it.
When it has cooled just enough to touch, squeeze out some of the
excess water.
Place the compress on your kidney area (the lower back)
and wrap it with a blanket or towel.
Sit with the compress on your back until it cools, then repeat once more.
Keep the kidney area warm all day.

In traditional Chinese medicine, the kidney area is where cold enters and leaves
the body. Ginger is a wonderful way to rewarm the body and increase the
circulation of your warm blood.

Wash your hands

Winter is paradise for germs.
Pay particular attention to your hand-washing today.
A good rule of thumb is to lather, wash and dry
in the time that it takes to sing the entire Happy
Birthday song.

It is so basic, but hand-washing is still our very best
frontline defence against colds, flu and other infections.
You have to do it well for it to be effective, so take the
time today to hone your hand-washing skills and keep
the winter bugs at bay.

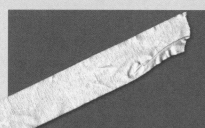

Herbal cream for aching joints

The cold of winter can make joints ache,
even in a young and active body.
If you have a winter ache, keep the affected joints warm and
rub on some arnica cream, some green-lipped mussel oil or
use a fresh ginger compress to ease the pain.

Green-lipped mussels are sea creatures that come from Marlborough Sound in
New Zealand. Numerous studies have found that they have an anti-inflammatory
action and so can help to reduce joint pain. Products made from the mussels are
now widely available from health food shops—look for reputable brands.

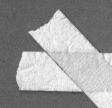

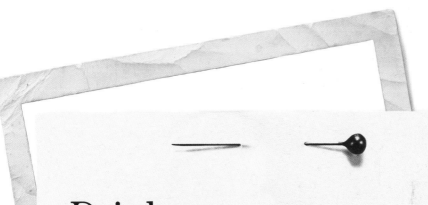

Drink up

Buy a large bottle of water.
Throughout the morning, drink it all.
In the afternoon, refill it and drink it again.

Our bodies are 55–75 per cent water and we need water for nearly every major bodily function. Dehydration (even 1–2 per cent) can cause symptoms such as dizziness, headache, poor concentration and coordination and it slows the metabolism. Two litres (3½ pints) of water a day helps keep you well hydrated.

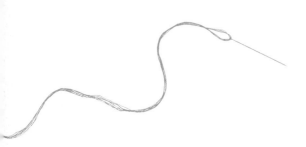

Clear your mind

What is one job you have been meaning to do for ages? It may be cleaning the oven, paying a bill, setting up a direct debit, calling family, sorting out the linen press. Find the time to do the job today.

All of these little jobs, mundane or not, sit in our minds and clutter it up. Slowly getting through these nagging jobs helps to clear the mind and gives us more energy and headspace to deal with life's everyday stresses. Often they sit in our minds for ages and only take ten minutes to finish when we actually get around to doing them.

Lost your mojo?

If you're having one of those days when you are feeling a bit flat and have lost your drive, get yourself some Dynamis Essence from a health food shop or chemist today and dose up.
It will help to recentre you and renew your enthusiasm for life.

An Australian naturopath, Ian White, spent many years researching and developing a range of native Australian Bush Flower Essences which are now widely available. Like the Bach flower essences, they work on a vibrational level to gently rebalance us. Australian Aborigines have used flowers to heal emotional imbalances and physical injuries for thousands of years, so it is great that we can now tap into this natural healing power.

Stretch it

Work out a two-minute stretch routine.
Involve your legs, arms, shoulders, neck, torso and bottom.
Just a few simple moves.
When you get out of bed each morning, do your two-minute routine before anything else.

As well as toning and lengthening, stretching gets the blood moving, the oxygen flowing and the energy surging. It is an easy way to get your mind, body and spirit ready to start a new day.

No, no, no

Do you ever say no to people?
If you don't have the time or energy to take on extra work,
practise saying no to people today.

Saying no is very hard for most people. We give and
give to others, but at the end of the day, have nothing
left for ourselves. It's ok to say no and keep some time
and energy for yourself. With some determination
and practice, you will find it easier to say a firm, but
gracious, no.

Naturally pain-free

If you suffer from aches and pains such as period pain, restless legs or crampy muscles, buy some Mag Phos Nerve and Muscle Relaxant today to pop into your natural first aid kit.

It's the tissue salt that's excellent for spasms, pains and cramps and a great one to try before a pharmaceutical pain-relief pill.

Start dosing, as per the instructions on the label, at the first sign of symptoms.

Tissue salts are simple, effective remedies that have been used since the nineteenth century. They are cheap and very low dose, so are safe for the whole family. You can buy them in a chewable tablet form or a lactose-free spray.

Stress backwards

Put your stress in reverse today.
Lie on the floor with your knees raised and your lower legs resting on a lounge or sofa.
Place a pillow under your head and a folded towel under your shoulder area.
Lie there for fifteen minutes.
Every few minutes, gently pull your chin in as if you are trying to push it into the floor.
Hold each tuck for a count of three, then relax.

This is a lovely gentle relaxation exercise which helps to relieve or reverse stress and also strengthen the neck.

Witchy winter brew

The chilly winter has been upon us for a while and it's time to make a warming brew, which herbalists call a decoction—sounds very witchy.

In a saucepan, add 1 stick cinnamon broken into small pieces, a 2 centimetre (1 inch) piece fresh ginger, finely chopped, and 1½ cups water.

Cover with a tightly fitting lid, bring to the boil then simmer for ten minutes.

Strain, add some honey or pure maple syrup if you wish to sweeten it, and drink it.

Cinnamon is a warming digestive and stimulates circulation. It helps to clear the nose and the lungs. Ginger is also good for digestion, helps you to relax and relieves nausea. This drink will warm your whole system.

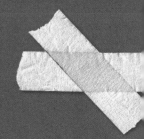

Winter tea

Bancha tea is the perfect tea for the colder months. It improves circulation, aids digestion, builds the blood and warms your body.
Get some today at the health food store.
Place a teaspoon in your cup, pour boiling water over it and allow to steep.
Sip and feel warm from the inside.

Bancha tea is also called Twig tea, kukicha or sannen bancha ('third year tea') as it is the twigs of the green tea plant harvested in their third year. It is virtually caffeine-free and is rich in the bone-building mineral calcium.

Slippers

Oh, there is nothing like a pair of comfy slippers on these cold winter nights. Nurture yourself and buy yourself a nice comfy pair today.

By nature, women are nurturers, but we don't often get nurtured ourselves. Doing little things for yourself can help you feel special and valued.

Carb down

Have a no-starchy-carbohydrate-day today.
Starchy carbohydrates are foods such as potato,
bread, biscuits, cake, anything made with grains
such as wheat, barley, oats, rye, rice or corn.

Having a day with no starchy carbohydrates makes you realise how
dependent your diet is on them. Reducing them in your diet is not only
great for weight loss, it can also boost your energy and encourage you
to increase the variety in your diet.

Girls' stuff

We need to have a pap smear every two years.
When was your last one?
Check your diary to see if you are due for another.
If you don't have a record, give your doctor a call today
to check.
Your GP can put you on the Pap Test Register to have a
reminder sent out to you every two years. A great list to
get on.

Time goes by so fast that it is hard to remember something every two years.
Pap smears are a vital part of health management, whether you are sexually
active or not. Although they cause a moment's discomfort, they save lives,
so ensure you put it in your diary, or get on a reminder list today.

Vegie boost

Today is Vegie Day.
Eat vegetables for every meal of the day.
Perhaps a carrot juice for breakfast, a warm salad for lunch
and roast vegetables for dinner.
Tomorrow you will reap the benefits.

Vegetables are high in nutritional goodies. Making one day each
week Vegie Day is a great way to boost your weekly intake, keep your
bowels moving and give your body a multivitamin treat.

Change your vocab

Remove three words from your vocabulary today.
The words are 'should', 'must' and 'ought'.
Don't let yourself use them at all for today.

The words 'should', 'must' and 'ought' evoke feelings of guilt, resentment and inadequacy. If they are part of your self-talk, the associated feelings may arise within you. If you use them toward others, these feelings will rise in them. Just eliminating these three words can help you express yourself in a more positive way and make a wonderful contribution to your emotional health.

A relaxed home

Take two minutes this morning to set up the oil burner with some relaxing essential oils.
Use a relaxation blend or your own blend.
Lavender, geranium and juniper are lovely for anxiety.
Neroli and bergamot are gentle and soothing.

Aromatherapy is a quick and easy way to change the energy in your home. Blending your own oils is a great way to get the exact benefits you are looking for. Everyone will associate the blend with you, and the safe, secure feeling of being home.

Fibre drive

Have at least two high-fibre foods at each meal today.
Choose one from the soluble and one from the insoluble
fibre lists below.
Good sources of soluble fibre include fruits, vegetables, oat
bran, barley, seed husks, flaxseed, psyllium, dried beans,
lentils, peas, soy milk and soy products.
Good sources of insoluble fibre include wheat bran, corn
bran, rice bran, the skins of fruits and vegetables, nuts,
seeds, dried beans and wholegrain foods.

A key role of fibre is to keep you regular, but it also has many other
fantastic functions in the body so even if you are already regular, a
fibre boost is great for your health. It can reduce blood cholesterol,
assist with weight control and help to stabilise blood sugars. When
boosting your fibre intake, it is very important to drink at least
2 litres (3½ pints) of water a day.

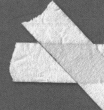

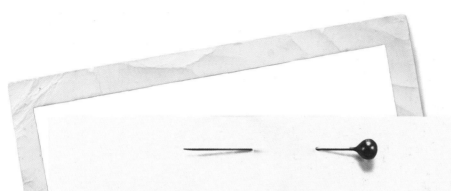

Melting moment

Run a warm bath.
Add 2 cups of Epsom salts.
Soak for twenty minutes.
You'll feel great!
The day will melt away and the weekend will seem that little bit closer.

Epsom salts, or magnesium sulphate, is a very cheap, old-fashioned naturopathic remedy. First produced in the town of Epsom, England, they are all natural and used for everything from soothing sore and tired muscles to detoxifying the body and natural haircare. When made into a poultice, they are also great for drawing out a splinter.

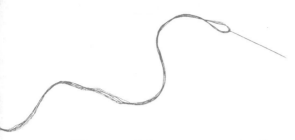

Dealing with pain

Got any aches or pains?
Is your lower back a bit sore, your neck stiff or your
legs aching?
Aches and pains can have a huge impact on your
quality of life and energy levels. Look into some
options for natural pain management.
Do some research today on herbalism, osteopathy,
physiotherapy, acupuncture or Bowen therapy and
take some positive steps to manage your aches
and pains.

Bowen therapy was developed more than 60 years ago. It focuses on the
gentle manipulation and release of the soft tissue or fascia. This stimulates
the body's receptors and enables the body to correct dysfunctions of
malalignments, thereby easing pain and discomfort.

Spring skin in winter

Make this oil blend for your bath tonight and wake up with beautiful spring skin tomorrow.
Blend 4 drops chamomile essential oil, 4 drops geranium essential oil and 2 drops patchouli essential oil with 1 tablespoon milk.
Add to the bath and soak.

Winter is hard on our skin. The cold, harsh weather can leave it feeling coarse, dry and scaly. This oil blend will restore it and leave it feeling soft and supple.

Caffeine-free day

Avoid caffeine today.
Try something new to drink.

Caffeine artificially stimulates and dehydrates the body, so give your body a complete rest occasionally. Try a fruit smoothie, fresh juice or a wheatgrass shot to give you the zip you get from caffeine.

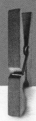

Fix it

Think of one nagging, menial but incredibly annoying problem or issue you have.
It may be cleaning the toilet, dirty socks left on the bathroom floor or deciding what's for dinner.
Find a way to fix it today.

Even small problems can add up to become major issues and impact on our wellbeing if left unchecked. If the timing is right, most people are willing to compromise and help you out with an issue you face. It may be giving the kids a star on their chart for putting their socks in the laundry, getting a house cleaner or sharing dinner cooking with your partner or flatmates. Address it while the issue is small and manageable.

Steam clean

Give your face a steam today to cleanse your skin and clear your nose.
Add 4 drops lavender essential oil and 3 drops eucalyptus oil or Breathe Easy to a pan of boiling water. Carefully place the pan onto a non-slip mat on a table. Hold your face about 40 centimetres (15 inches) from the hot pan and place a towel over your head.
Close your eyes and breathe in the lovely steam for 5–10 minutes.

We are halfway through winter. For most of us, our skin and our sinuses are suffering a little by this time of year. Steaming is an excellent way to clear both. It also stimulates circulation and hydrates the skin. If you have dry or sensitive skin, don't steam more than once a fortnight.

Leg rest

While you are washing the dishes, waiting in line,
standing at work or doing any activity that involves
standing for a prolonged period today,
put one leg on a higher level.
You could rest it on a shelf, a step or the rung of a stool.

Changing the level of your feet helps to support and reduce strain
on your back.

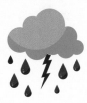

Face it

Have a good look at your face.
In India's ancient ayurvedic medicine, horizontal wrinkling on the forehead shows deep-seated anxieties and worries. Puffiness under the eyes can indicate that the kidneys need some support.
A vertical line between the eyebrows on the left-hand side can indicate suppressed emotions in the spleen. A line on the right-hand side shows suppressed emotions in the liver.

Our bodies are constantly communicating with us, through changes in our faces, hair, nails, tongues, etc. We need to become attuned to our body, and act before we fall into illness or imbalance. Facial diagnosis is used extensively as part of the ayurvedic system of medicine which has been practised since the ancient Vedic period (1–6 century BCE). The face is the mirror of the mind in this system of medicine, and imbalance, disorders and disease are reflected on the face in the form of wrinkles, lines and marks. The face is used as a key diagnostic tool. If you are interested, go online and do some research on Vedic face diagnosis and ayurvedic medicine.

Sore tummy tea

If someone in the house has woken with a sore tummy today, try this gentle tea.
Make a pot of green tea and add 5 green cardamom pods.
Allow to steep for five minutes and serve with honey if desired.

This soothing tea is from Pakistan and is wonderful for helping sore or upset stomachs.

Watch your mouth

Listen to your mind's chatter today.
We talk to ourselves endlessly in our mind, but how much of it is positive?
Often repeated self-defeating phrases—like 'I'm so stupid' or 'I never get that right'—start to become real in our minds, much like a self-fulfilling prophecy, so begin to consciously answer back and reprogram yourself.
Try some positive affirmations or statements, so instead of 'I can't do this', say 'I am confident and brave. I will do this.'
Write down your positive affirmations and leave them somewhere you can read them often.
Get them firmly imbedded in your mind so they can begin to unseat the negatives.

There is great power in negative self-talk. It can be a very destructive force if left unchecked. Being conscious of what we say about ourselves can help to unlock old patterns of thought and negative self-images.

Banish the winter blues

Even the happiest among us can get a little down in the middle of winter.
Try these natural mood lifters today to bring some sunshine back into your life.
Get some natural light, go for a walk or do some exercise, limit your stress and boost your good-mood foods. These include lean animal and plant protein, seeds, nuts, green leafy vegetables, deep-sea fish, flaxseed and sprouts.

The major 'happy' messengers in the body are serotonin and adrenaline. Put simply, serotonin helps mood and adrenaline helps motivation. An imbalance in either can lead to low mood, poor motivation, lack of concentration, behaviour problems or poor sleep, to name just a few. Both are made from protein and helped along by the good-mood foods listed above.
Diet, exercise and natural light can really help to lift your mood and spirits even on the darkest winter days.

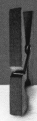

Pee control

Do five sets of pelvic floor exercises every time you see a traffic light today.
Imagine you need to do a wee but have to hold on.
These muscles are your pelvic floor muscles.
Tighten the muscles and hold for five seconds.
Remember the 'five for five' rule—five repeats held for five seconds each.

A strong set of pelvic floor muscles means you won't need to run to the loo at a minute's notice, cross your legs before your sneeze or ask people to warn you before they tell a joke! It can also do wonders for your sex life. . .

Smile

Smile at three strangers today.

It is easy, free and it just makes you
and them feel great.

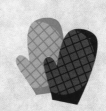

Congestion buster

Some time during winter, chances are someone in your family will be congested so take five minutes this morning to make some thyme and ginger tea. Place 2 tablespoons freshly chopped thyme in a small saucepan with a knob of grated ginger. Add water and bring to the boil, then place in a teapot to steep for five minutes. Add honey to taste. Sip the warm tea throughout the day.

Thyme is antiseptic and helps soothe colds and sore throats, while ginger helps to break down mucus. If possible, use Manuka honey, as this sweetens the tea and has its own wonderful medicinal properties.

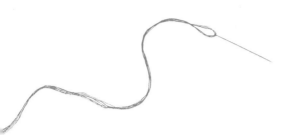

Sleep tight

Set yourself up for a sound sleep. If you have children, ask your partner to get up for them tonight, so you can have a solid, restorative sleep.

For a sound sleep, develop a relaxing bedtime routine. Have a warm cup of herbal tea or milk, take a bath, sit quietly for a few minutes to clear your mind, or listen to some soothing music. Avoid stimulants such as caffeine and sugar. Turn off the TV and computer.

Sound sleep is pivotal to your wellbeing. It is not always possible when you have young children, but by sharing the load, at least one night a week, you can have a solid sleep which will do wonders for your wellbeing.

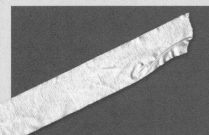

Be naturally sweet

Replace your sugar today with a more healthful alternative. Try some barley malt syrup in your tea, stevia on your cereal or pure maple syrup in your milkshake.

Reducing the white sugar in your diet has some excellent health benefits but does not mean you can't have something sweet. There are many natural alternatives that have their own nutritional benefits. Barley malt syrup, apple and pear juice concentrate, pure maple syrup and dates are all super sweet and are rich in nutrients. Check out the alternatives in your supermarket or health food shop.

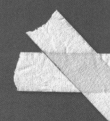

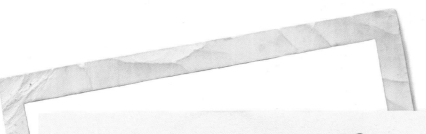

Treasure chest

No, we're not being pirates today
but we are making a treasure chest.
Choose a few things that are special to you.
It may be some letters, jewellery, small gifts,
anything that is significant.
Place them in a box with some tissue paper
and tie it up with a ribbon.
Keep it in a private place where only you will find it.
Take it out when you feel you need some time to reconnect
with yourself.

Spending time with your treasures can help to remind you of who you are, who
cares for you and where you have been. It can help to lift you out of current
circumstances by giving you a wider perspective on your life and loves.

A warm way to start the day

Have porridge for breakfast today. Eat it warm with a drizzle of honey and chopped nuts.

Oats are a wonderful tonic for busy women. They calm the nerves, and relieve tension, anxiety and exhaustion. They have a sweet, warm quality and so are the perfect winter breakfast.

Kidney warmers

Keep your kidneys protected from the winter cold and they will keep you protected from winter ills.

Your kidneys are an entry and exit for temperature in the body. They are vulnerable in the cold of winter and need to be kept warm. The kidneys can be found directly above your hip bones on your back (those fat pads are there to protect them). Wear a warm woolly jumper today or a top that pulls down over the top of your trousers, and you won't regret it.

Say it out loud

Today, choose five people in your life you are close to.
Tell each of them three things you love about them.

Sometimes we need to take a minute to appreciate what we have,
to be grateful for the people in our lives who enrich it and make
us feel valued and loved. Take some time today to tell them what
they mean to you.

Nutrient table

Nutrient	Great sources
Vitamin A	apricots, carrots, green leafy vegetables, egg yolk, broccoli, sweet potato
Vitamin B group	legumes, wheatgerm, whole grains, avocado, eggs, broccoli, salmon, chicken, meat, green vegetables, mushrooms
Vitamin B6	chicken, egg yolk, legumes, oatmeal, salmon, tuna, walnuts
Vitamin C	broccoli, blackcurrants, citrus fruits, peas, cabbage, kiwi, guava, sweet potato, berries, strawberries
Vitamin E	almonds, beef, corn, eggs, rye, oats, nuts, wheatgerm
Omega 3	pepitas, linseed (flaxseed) oil, sunflower seeds, walnuts, salmon, tuna, cod
Calcium	almonds, broccoli, buckwheat, dairy, figs, egg yolk, green leafy vegetables
Chromium	asparagus, apples, egg yolk, potatoes, mushrooms, nuts
Iodine	lima beans, mushrooms, oysters, sunflower seeds, cod
Magnesium	almonds, cashews, molasses, parsnips, soy beans, whole grains, eggs, seeds
Zinc	cashews, beef, egg yolk, milk, sunflower seeds, pepitas, whole grains